Depression

YOUR QUESTIONS ANSWERED

D1585965

For Elsevier

Commissioning Editor: Fiona Conn
Project Development Manager: Fiona Conn, Isobel Black
Project Manager: Frances Affleck
Designer: George Ajayi
Illustration Manager: Bruce Hogarth
Illustrator: John Marshall

Depression

YOUR QUESTIONS ANSWERED

Cosmo Hallström
MB CHB FRCP FRCPSYCH
Formerly Consultant Psychiatrist, Charing Cross Hospital;
Honorary Senior Lecturer, Imperial College Medical School,
London, UK

Nicola McClure
MBBS MRCS LRCP
Principal in General Practice, Shepherds Bush, London, UK

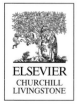

ELSEVIER
CHURCHILL
LIVINGSTONE

EDINBURGH LONDON NEW YORK OXFORD PHILADELPHIA ST LOUIS SYDNEY TORONTO 2005

ELSEVIER
CHURCHILL
LIVINGSTONE

First published 2005

ISBN 0 4330 7290 6

British Library Cataloguing in Publication Data
A catalogue record for this book is available from the British Library

Library of Congress Cataloging in Publication Data
A catalog record for this book is available from the Library of Congress

Note
Medical knowledge is constantly changing. Standard safety precautions must be followed, but as new research and clinical experience broaden our knowledge, changes in treatment and drug therapy may become necessary or appropriate. Readers are advised to check the most current product information provided by the manufacturer of each drug to be administered to verify the recommended dose, the method and duration of administration, and contraindications. It is the responsibility of the practitioner, relying on experience and knowledge of the patient, to determine dosages and the best treatment for each individual patient. Neither the Publisher nor the authors assume any liability for any injury and/or damage to persons or property arising from this publication.
The Publisher

ELSEVIER your source for books,
journals and multimedia
in the health sciences

www.elsevierhealth.com

The
Publisher's
policy is to use
**paper manufactured
from sustainable forests**

Contents

Preface

Depression is one of the commonest conditions family doctors will encounter and is often treated entirely within the primary-care setting. With modern treatments, both medical and psychological, we are now able to offer patients much more, and there is increasing awareness that depression is a very treatable condition. Indeed it is important to treat depression early and intensively to prevent chronicity and to alleviate the undoubted misery and morbidity it causes.

This book follows a simple question-and-answer format. The questions are asked by a practising GP and the answers supplied by a consultant psychiatrist, the two having worked together for nearly twenty years. We aim to offer practical advice on the sort of problems seen in the surgery nearly every day. Much of the book comprises advice not found in the standard textbooks, which often concentrate on theory and not on the sort of management problems that beset GPs in busy surgeries.

Although the book is aimed primarily at GPs, it should also be of value to other professionals involved in the day-to-day care of depressed patients – psychiatric nurses, psychologists and social workers – to help them understand the thinking that goes on in the management of depression. It may also be of value to patients and their families and help to unravel some of the medical mystique that may surround their problem and its treatment. In doing so it should help them to become more involved in their treatment, thereby speeding up their recovery.

Cosmo Hallström
Nicki McClure

How to use this book

The *Your Questions Answered* series aims to meet the information needs of GPs and other primary care professionals who care for patients with chronic conditions. It is designed to help them work with patients and their families, providing effective, evidence-based care and management.

The books are in an accessible question and answer format, with detailed contents lists at the beginning of every chapter and a complete index to help find specific information.

ICONS

Icons are used in the book to identify particular types of information:

 highlights information important to clinical practice

 highlights side effect information

 highlights case studies which illustrate or help to explain the answers given

PATIENT QUESTIONS

At the end of relevant chapters there are sections of frequently asked patient questions, with easy-to-understand answers aimed at the non-medical reader. These questions are also listed at the end of the book.

What is depression?

1

1.1 Is depression a new concept?

The concept of melancholia (black bile) was mentioned in texts of Hippocrates. Subsequently, attempts to explain mental illness in somatic terms vied with the theological interpretation that melancholy was a consequence of sin. In the 18th and 19th centuries, concepts of melancholy concentrated on the symptomatology rather than the causation. Gradually, during this period, humane treatments and attitudes to insanity began to develop.

The modern concepts of depression evolved towards the end of the 19th century when depressive illnesses were seen as distinct from other forms of mental illness, such as dementia praecox (schizophrenia) and general paralysis of the insane. The modern classifications derive from this, although concentrating initially on the severe end of the spectrum where the patients were in institutional care. The final stage in the recognition of depressive disorders has come about since the Second World War as a result of a liberalization of society and increased access to health care. More importantly, the use of electroconvulsive therapy (ECT) in the treatment of depression and the development of effective antidepressants made it a worthwhile task to seek out patients with depression and to provide effective treatments at an early stage, before the conditions became chronic. Associated with this has been a gradual destigmatization of mental illness in general and depression in particular.

Thus after the introduction of imipramine, in 1957, and of the monoamine oxidase inhibitor (MAOI) isoniazid, in 1958, treatment became available for patients who previously had spent prolonged periods in mental hospitals. The success with the more severe end of the spectrum encouraged treatment of patients with the less severe disorders. The development of antidepressants with less debilitating side-effects, increased access to information and higher patient expectations have resulted in greater awareness, recognition and treatment of depression. More recently there has been increasing interest in the social and psychological antecedents of depressive illness.

The latest phase in our thinking about depression and its treatment concentrates on issues such as the quality of life of patients receiving treatment and the problem of side-effects, which is especially important if patients are to be treated in the long term to prevent relapses when they are effectively well. Side-effects may be acceptable when treating severe illness, but not so when the patient is on long-term treatment and without current problems.

Other current issues include cost–benefit analysis of treatments in financial terms. Modern antidepressants have become victims of their own success, attracting a backlash of some popular opinion, which complains about over-medicalizing unhappiness and voices concerns about dependency, withdrawal and even suicidality as a result of antidepressant treatment.

Perhaps the most important therapeutic issue remains the low rate of success of the treatment of depression compared with modern treatments of other mental illnesses, which are about 70% effective (depending on how that is measured). A significant proportion of patients suffering from this common condition do not become cured, leaving a large number of patients who remain unwell in the long term, despite the best interventions of their therapists. Little is heard about this unfortunate group.

1.2 How would you describe depression?

Depression is a broad concept. For our purposes it is a condition characterized by pathologically low mood. It embodies a broad spectrum of conditions, with unhappiness at one end of the spectrum and severe 'endogenous' biological-type mood disorders at the other end. From a medical point of view, depression is an illness characterized by a series of depressive symptoms with prescribed treatments. There are other ways of defining it according to sociological, existential and psychological views.

1.3 What is the difference between depression and unhappiness?

The difference between unhappiness and depression is both qualitative and quantitative. The severity of the symptoms and their chronicity are important. Depression tends to be more severe and longer lasting. It is also a question of state and trait. Trait is a long-term personality factor that tends to remain relatively constant throughout life. States vary according to situations and internal and external factors. Some people are born pessimists and carry the world's burdens on their shoulders. They may be regarded as having a depressive personality, or dysthymia. Unhappiness is generally understandable in psychological or environmental terms. In depression the response is often out of proportion to the circumstances.

There is obviously a large degree of overlap. The diagnosis of depression relies more on the medical model, with reference to internal mechanisms and a certain lack of individual control of the situation. It implies a disease. Unhappiness suggests a more holistic view of the situation with a greater degree of personal responsibility of the victim and a more psychological model.

1.4 What predisposes people to depressive illness?

Some people react better to adverse situations and therefore do not succumb to depression very easily, while others do not seem to have the emotional wherewithal to cope and they become depressed easily. The key to this lies in individual variability and vulnerability. It is also an interaction between nature and nurture. Vulnerability factors include a genetic predisposition. Other biological variables suggest that people are susceptible to developing depression at certain periods in their lives and not at others; some become depressed even in the absence of an adequate stimulus.

Psychological predeterminants affect the individual's learned ability to react to stress. People who have learned to be more self-assured and to cope with stress are less likely to develop depression when challenged than those who have learned to cope poorly or see change as a threat rather than an opportunity. There is also the question of the nature of the adverse situation. For example, the loss of a parent may have a major impact on someone who continues to live in the family home, whereas it may have much less impact if that person has not seen that parent for 20 years.

1.5 Is there a genetic basis for depression?

A strong genetic basis for the inheritance of severe depressive illness has been demonstrated in the study of twins. Identical twins, separated at birth, have a high concordance of about 70% for depression, and dizygotic twins have a lower concordance rate of about 20%. The risk of depression is about 10% if one parent has a history and about 20% if both parents are affected, as opposed to a risk of 1–2% if there is no family history. As a clinician I often see depression running in families in which a parent, grandparent or uncle or aunt also have the illness. The more the condition moves away from the classic bipolar mood disorder towards the clinical picture of 'reactive depression' or unhappiness, the less important is the genetic component.

1.6 To what extent can depression be considered a learned behaviour?

An element of learned behaviour is involved; inheritance is not sufficient to account for all causes of depression. Learned helplessness, learning from our parents, and the way we learn to see and experience the world will influence our psychological vulnerability. Psychoanalytical theories also provide an insight into subconscious influences on our perceptions of loss and depression. Those with a pessimistic view of the world will project a negative interpretation of events.

1.7 More women attend surgery with symptoms of depression, but does this reflect the true distribution of the condition?

Overall, depressive disorders are twice as common in women. Bipolar affective disorder, however, is equally common amongst men and women. The highest prevalence rate for depressive disorders is in women between 35 and 45 years. In men the prevalence rate increases with age. The overall prevalence rate is 3–4% of the general population. It is more common amongst divorced and separated people. Men often have their depression diagnosed as problems with alcohol or personality problems. They often project their suffering outwards. Women are culturally more allowed to express their suffering and thereby to present to doctors. There may also be a sex-linked inheritance that makes the genetic loading for depression greater among women, although this is not certain. (*See also Qs 4.43 and 4.44.*)

1.8 How does deprivation affect depression?

There is a strong deprivation gradient – the highest prevalence of depression is found in the most deprived category – not only for depression but also anxiety, coronary heart disease and type 2 diabetes. Middle-aged people also have poorer outcomes, especially women with heart disease and men with depression. Social deprivation is bad for your health generally.

1.9 What is the biochemical basis for depression?

The predominant view – 'the amine hypothesis of depression' – is that there is a functional deficiency in one or more of three amine neurotransmitter systems. These are 5HT (5-hydroxytryptamine or serotonin), dopamine and noradrenaline. This theory has stood the test of time, but is too simplistic to describe the full situation. One major drawback to the amine theory is that antidepressants exert their pharmacological action within minutes or hours, but it is well established that the therapeutic response takes several weeks, so there must be a time-dependent component in the mechanism of antidepressant action.

Reduced levels of dopamine may be the mechanism for reduced psychomotor activity in depression and elevated activity in mania. The most widely implicated neurotransmitter is 5HT. Reduced levels can cause depression. Most antidepressants and anti-anxiety drugs have an effect of increasing 5HT activity. Other mechanisms are also involved. Acetylcholine may be important, but its role has not fully been explored. New neurotransmitters, such as 'substance P' and pregabalin, exert an effect in mood regulation, and their roles are being explored in depression.

The above-mentioned neurotransmitters work at the synapse between nerve cells. There is now considerable interest in second messenger systems, which act after the synaptic receptor in the generation of nerve impulses. The integration of the functioning of these separate neuronal systems is also important because each neurotransmitter system closely interacts with the others, and it is often impossible to say where the primary disturbance lies and to try to disentangle what is a primary phenomenon and what is a secondary effect in the control of mood. It is a very difficult area to understand because of the inaccessibility of the depressed human brain to chemical analysis.

1.10 Do hydrocortisone levels affect mood?

Many patients with depression have elevated hydrocortisone levels and loss of the circadian cycle. This may be a measure of stress or a function of depression itself. Half of patients with severe depression fail to suppress endogenous hydrocortisone levels after receiving dexamethasone – this is the basis of the dexamethasone suppression test, a weak biological marker for depression.

Hormonal abnormalities often cause a mood disturbance. Patients treated with cortisone or those with Cushing's disease may become depressed. Other patients on steroids can acquire an elevated mood. Steroids may also be involved in the way that antidepressants and neurotransmitters bind to receptors. It would appear that the relationship between hydrocortisone and mood is intimate but non-specific. There are many endocrine abnormalities in depression. Hormonal release is under the control of the mood-regulating neurotransmitters 5HT and dopamine.

1.11 What does neuroimaging have to tell us about depression?

Structural abnormalities on CT scanning have been demonstrated in older patients with depression – these are mainly enlarged ventricles and reduced brain substance. Subcortical hyperintensities can be shown on MRI in white matter and basal ganglia in depressed patients. Reduction in activity in the prefrontal and cingulate cortex can be shown with functional neuroimaging.

More recently it has been shown that external psychological stressors, such as those found in post-traumatic stress disorders can cause structural changes in the brain. This reinforces the notion of the biological impact of psychological factors on structure and function. Some cases of depression can quite clearly be shown to have a biological basis. The field of neuroimaging is evolving rapidly and shows great promise in helping our understanding of how the brain malfunctions in depression.

1.12 Do you think that there is still some sort of stigma attached to the diagnosis of depression? I ask this because lots of patients prefer to have the word 'stress' written on their medical certificates rather than 'depression'.

Sadly there is a widespread stigma against all mental illness and all mental disability. A diagnosis of stress implies outside causative factors. Depression implies some form of personal vulnerability, weakness or instability – physical disability is seen as more acceptable. Patients fear discrimination and stigmatization by their employers and colleagues. A Royal College of Psychiatrists' survey revealed that people had difficulties defining depression. They thought it could run in families; it could be caused by bereavements, redundancy and other external factors. The public is generally sympathetic to depression. The majority considered a GP to be the best person to deal with it. Counselling was generally seen as the treatment of choice.

For more information on stigmatization of mental illness and discrimination against those suffering from it, see the Royal College of Psychiatrists' 'Changing Minds' campaign at www.changingminds.co.uk.

1.13 It is said that we only deal with the 'tip of the iceberg' when we treat depression. If this is so, what proportion remains undiagnosed and untreated and why?

Depression is one of the most common conditions a GP will treat: it affects 3% of the population at any one time. A GP will recognize and treat about half of the patients who present to him with depression (*see Box 1.1*). The other half will have 'masked depression', which may not be recognized. Of these diagnosed patients, only about one in ten will be referred on to a specialist. The majority of depressive illnesses are dealt with by the GP. Cases in young men under 30 are particularly likely to be missed.

The statistics are heavily dependent upon the threshold for diagnosing depression, but depression in its wider sense is so widespread that doctors almost don't see the wood for the trees. It presents in all manner of ways, such as excessive concern about either minor ailments (somatization syndrome), chronic pain syndromes, delayed recovery from other illnesses, and excess drinking and smoking. GPs have become increasingly aware of issues surrounding depression as a result of initiatives such as the 'Defeat Depression Campaign', which ran from 1992 to 1996, more accessible treatments and increased public awareness. Recent campaigns have included Mind's 'Mind Out for Mental Health' and, in Scotland, the 'See Me' anti-stigma campaign.

A major barrier preventing patients consulting their GP for their depression is the thought that GPs just hand out pills, and that the GP is too busy.

BOX 1.1 Prevalence of depression, and proportions treated in primary and secondary care

- 3% of the community are depressed
- 75% of these patients present to the GP
- 60% are diagnosed and treated by the GP
- 5% are referred to a specialist
- 0.5% are admitted to hospital

1.14 Are the old terms 'endogenous' and 'exogenous depression' still used and do they have any relevance?

They are no longer parts of the standard ICD-10 (*International Classification of Diseases*, 10th edn, published by the World Health Organization) and DSM-IV (*Diagnostic and Statistical Manual of Mental Disorders*, 4th edn, published by the American Psychiatric Association) systems that dominate the modern classifications. The general view is that most psychiatric disorders are multifactorial in causation: external factors impinge on internal vulnerability factors. Modern psychiatric classification relies upon the description of the condition rather than its causation. It describes the clinical picture. The exceptions to this are post-traumatic stress disorders and adjustment disorders, in which the causation is included in the diagnosis. If the condition is clearly caused by external factors then the diagnosis will be adjustment disorder with a depressive reaction. It is accepted that life-events can trigger a depressive reaction. The widely used DSM-IV diagnostic system applies the concept of 'axes' to quantify vulnerability factors such as personality and external stressors (*Box 1.2*).

1.15 What is the peak age for a depressive illness?

The answer is complicated. The mean age of onset for bipolar illnesses is generally seen as about 21. General neurotic-type depression is related to unhappiness, and social adversity is also more common in young people. Once established, major depressive illness tends to recur, and the prevalence of depression increases with age to a maximum in the 35 to 45 age group (*see Table 1.1*). Other factors then become important in the manifestation of depression – notably social factors such as unemployment, redundancy, divorce and separation, and social isolation and ill-health – factors which are more influential with increasing age. On the other hand, as people mature, the volatility of personality diminishes and they become better at developing coping strategies, which have a protective function. As can be seen from *Table 1.1*, there is a counterintuitive decrease in lifetime prevalence rates after the mid-life peak. The explanation may lie in earlier death of depressed people, worsening memory for previous depressions, or a real change in rates of depression in different birth cohorts.

BOX 1.2 DSM-IV axes

Axis I:	the clinical disorder
Axis II:	personality factors
Axis III:	general medical conditions
Axis IV:	psychosocial and environmental factors
Axis V:	a global assessment of function

TABLE 1.1 Prevalence of depression by age group		
Age (years)	Lifetime prevalence	One-year prevalence
18–29	7%	4%
30–44	10%	5%
45–64	5%	3%
65+	2%	1.5%

1.16 Is there a danger that we are being encouraged by the drug industry to medicalize normal reactions to social situations, so creating a huge pool of mental ill-health that requires treatment?

This would be the view of a sociologist less interested in the practical realities of the welfare of a patient sitting in front of him. The critical issue is whether the individual who comes for help can be offered help. If social factors are important or relevant, they need to be addressed – although there is often no simple solution to poverty, social exclusion, personality disorder and relationship difficulties. Medication is unlikely to be very helpful, although it is sometimes worth a brief trial if social factors are to the fore. There is certainly a superficially attractive health-economics argument (and anti-medical-model position) to suggest that we are over-treating depression and that people who are not classically mentally ill should forget about doctors and seek help elsewhere. It may save time for the doctor and money from the drugs budget, but does not do a lot for the patient. The general view, borne out by the data, is that for every depressed patient treated by a GP there is another one whose condition goes unrecognized. The drug industry, which usually provides most interventions that GPs use in all therapeutic areas, suddenly becomes suspect when dealing with emotional problems, and I think this is a residue of the anti-psychiatric lobby of the 1960s and symptomatic of the industry being a victim of its own success. The huge pool of mental illness that requires treatment is a function of society's unmet need and increased expectations. These may in some ways be unrealistic, but the drug industry can hardly be blamed for that.

My main concern is that the treatments we have are sadly not that effective and we can only offer proper help to a proportion of our patients, which means that there is room for philosophical debate as to what to do with the remainder. Depression is under-diagnosed and under-treated. I believe that both doctors and the industry have a communality of purpose in raising the profile and needs of the depressed patient and providing an effective treatment if possible. The skill of the doctor is to decide who should be treated with medication and for how long.

1.17 How can I diagnose depression in the presence of physical illness?

When patients have physical illness we often forget that they can have emotional and even psychiatric problems associated with their illness and even independent of it. Doctors and patients tend to focus on the obvious problem and tend to gloss over the secondary issues such as mood disorders. Patients with serious physical illnesses often have mood disturbances that may be understandable or may be out of proportion to their problems. Chronic pain, serious illness and unexplained symptoms will quite reasonably cause anxiety and even depression in most patients. Whether this then responds to simple measures such as good healthcare and dealing with the physical problems, together with reassurance and support, or whether it needs specific psychiatric intervention, needs exploration. Often if the depression associated with physical illness is treated effectively, then the overall recovery or at least functional improvement of the physical illness is greater. Other conditions, such as stroke and chronic pain, are often associated with frank depressive illnesses and benefit from vigorous treatment of the depression. About 20% of patients who have had heart attacks become depressed; and depression independently increases the risk of development of subsequent strokes or heart attacks by some three- or four-fold (as important a factor as high cholesterol). So it is always worth looking out for depressive illness that can be treated in physically ill patients. If there is doubt, the Hospital Anxiety and Depression Scale (*see Q. 4.33*) is a useful screening instrument to see whether a patient has significant depressive symptoms worthy of further exploration. It has been validated to detect mood disorders in patients with physical illness. (*See also Qs 4.31 to 4.42.*)

PATIENT QUESTION

1.18 What causes depression?

The causes of depression are multiple, but they can be summed up as an interaction between an individual and the world around him or her. Depression is often caused by 'loss' – a bereavement or a breakdown in a relationship. It can result from multiple difficult life situations and problematic lifestyles. Difficult relationships, financial problems and social problems can all lead to a low mood. In addition, there is substantial personal vulnerability. Some people have an optimistic view of the world and deal with problems as they arise; others are more easily worn down. A lot of this is to do with how the individual has learned to see the world. Some people are born victims; others tend to rise above situations. Much of this attitude to life develops in childhood and at a very early age. Some see new situations as a threat rather than an opportunity. This view of the world is often learned from childhood expectations. In addition there is a 'constitutional element'. Some people are born to be unhappy and others not so, and the tendency often runs in families. So there are genetic, psychological, developmental and environmental–social factors that all interact.

The diagnosis of depression

2

2.1 What are the core symptoms of depression?

The symptoms in *Box 2.1* are the ones that most clearly identify the illness and are those most likely to change as a result of treatment. If three of these are present to a clinically significant degree, then the patient is probably depressed, and the presence of four or more should result in an appropriate treatment programme being established.

2.2 What are the physical symptoms of depression?

Poor sleep, especially with frequent waking during the night and early morning waking, is of diagnostic importance in depression. Loss of appetite, weight loss of as much as 5% of body weight per month and constipation are other indicative biological features of depression. Tiredness and lethargy and general psychomotor retardation are also indicative. Sometimes the converse is true, and patients have an increase in appetite, put on some weight and have hypersomnia. So these physical symptoms are of considerable diagnostic interest but are not pathognomonic of depression.

Patients may exhibit psychomotor retardation, with poverty of facial expression, sparse and slow speech and a general slowing of thinking, difficulty in formulating ideas and an inability to make decisions. Other patients may be agitated, with restlessness involving pacing, fidgeting and the same thought recurring constantly without any action being taken. Other features include a loss of libido with possible impotence or frigidity, muscle pains and difficulty coping with physical tasks at work.

2.3 What are the clinical signs of depression?

A sad face, reduced spontaneity of movement, paucity of gestures, poor eye-contact, poverty of speech, distractibility and signs of anxiety. Weight loss

---

BOX 2.1 Core symptoms of depression

■ Sadness
■ Loss of interest
■ Poor appetite
■ Sleep difficulty
■ Loss of energy
■ Pessimism or guilt
■ Suicidal ideation

may also be a physical sign of depression. These signs are not very reliable, however. Some patients can put on a stoical front, and many patients are on their best behaviour during a GP consultation.

2.4 How may depression present?

Not all depressed patients will tell you that they are depressed. Features in the history which suggest a diagnosis of depression are listed in Box 2.2.

The depression may be out of proportion to what could be expected from any stress occurring now or that the patient has previously endured. These features should make you consider the diagnosis, although other conditions, both mental and physical, can also result in similar complaints.

The DSM-IV criteria for a major depressive episode (*see Q. 3.1*) are given in *Box 2.3*, and those for specifying melancholic features (*see Q. 3.7*) in an episode are given in *Box 2.4*.

2.5 What is the Hamilton Depression Rating Scale?

This scale (*see Appendix 1*), devised by Max Hamilton in the late 1950s, is the most widely used depression rating scale in the world. It has become the benchmark scale in clinical trials, although there are arguably better scales around. It appears to be clinically relevant and easy to understand, and it has stood the test of time. It assumes that the more symptoms the patient has and the worse they are, the worse the depression is overall. It should really be used to detect change more than as an absolute measure of severity, although it gives an indication of that, too. It has to be filled out by the doctors rather than the patient. A score of 0 to 7 is in the normal range; 8 to 17 indicates mild depression; 18 to 25 moderate depression; and over 26 shows severe depression.

BOX 2.2 Typical acute presentations of depression

- Normal activity disrupted: unable to cope with daily duties; unable to go to work; unable to get out of bed
- Vague physical symptoms: tiredness; loss of appetite and weight; insomnia
- Difficulty coping: alcohol abuse; drug abuse; violent impulses or behaviour
- Worried family and friends: frustration; loss of sympathy; guilt
- Suicidal thoughts, plans, attempts

BOX 2.3 DSM-IV criteria for major depressive episode

A. Five (or more) of the following symptoms have been present during the same 2-week period and represent a change from previous functioning; at least one of the symptoms is either (1) depressed mood or (2) loss of interest or pleasure:
(**Note:** Do not include symptoms that are clearly due to a general medical condition, or mood-incongruent delusions or hallucinations)
  (1) depressed mood most of the day, nearly every day, as indicated by either subjective report (e.g. feels sad or empty) or observation made by others (e.g. appears tearful). **Note:** In children and adolescents, can be irritable mood
  (2) markedly diminished interest or pleasure in all, or almost all, activities most of the day, nearly every day (as indicated by either subjective account or observation made by others)
  (3) significant weight loss when not dieting or weight gain (e.g., a change of more than 5% of body weight in a month), or decrease or increase in appetite nearly every day. **Note:** In children, consider failure to make expected weight gains
  (4) insomnia or hypersomnia nearly every day
  (5) psychomotor agitation or retardation nearly every day (observable by others, not merely subjective feelings of restlessness or being slowed down)
  (6) fatigue or loss of energy nearly every day
  (7) feelings of worthlessness or excessive or inappropriate guilt (which may be delusional) nearly every day (not merely self-reproach or guilt about being sick)
  (8) diminished ability to think or concentrate, or indecisiveness, nearly every day (either by subjective account or as observed by others)
  (9) recurrent thoughts of death (not just fear of dying), recurrent suicidal ideation without a specific plan, or a suicide attempt or a specific plan for committing suicide
B. The symptoms do not meet criteria for a mixed episode
C. The symptoms cause clinically significant distress or impairment in social, occupational, or other important areas of functioning
D. The symptoms are not due to the direct physiological effects of a substance (e.g. a drug of abuse, a medication) or a general medical condition (e.g. hypothyroidism)
E. The symptoms are not better accounted for by bereavement, i.e. after the loss of a loved one, the symptoms persist for longer than 2 months or are characterized by marked functional impairment, morbid preoccupation with worthlessness, suicidal ideation, psychotic symptoms, or psychomotor retardation

---

BOX 2.4 DSM-IV criteria for melancholic features

Specify if:

With melancholic features (can be applied to the current or most recent major depressive episode in major depressive disorder and to a major depressive episode in bipolar I or bipolar II disorder only if it is the most recent type of mood episode)

A. Either of the following, occurring during the most severe period of the current episode:
   (1) loss of pleasure in all, or almost all, activities
   (2) lack of reactivity to usually pleasurable stimuli (does not feel much better, even temporarily, when something good happens)

B. Three (or more) of the following:
   (1) distinct quality of depressed mood (i.e., the depressed mood is experienced as distinctly different from the kind of feeling experienced after the death of a loved one)
   (2) depression regularly worse in the morning
   (3) early morning awakening (at least 2 hours before usual time of awakening)
   (4) marked psychomotor retardation or agitation
   (5) significant anorexia or weight loss
   (6) excessive or inappropriate guilt

Reprinted with permission from the Diagnostic and Statistical Manual of Mental Disorders, Text Revision, Copyright 2000. American Psychiatric Association.

2.6 In the surgery I have often found the GHQ a more useful tool – particularly as it is filled in by the patient. Have you any comment on this?

The General Health Questionnaire (GHQ) measures 'caseness' on a statistical probability, rather than depression itself. It applies to all forms of mental distress. As an instrument it is simple to administer and user-friendly and is amongst the best available tools to use as a screening instrument to detect 'cases'. It is filled out by the patient and so saves time for the doctor, and can also be used as a screening tool while the patient is waiting to be seen. Another useful instrument is the HADS (*see Q. 4.33*), which is specifically designed to screen for depression and anxiety in patients with a physical illness.

These are only screening instruments, and not a substitute for a proper history and examination of mental state.

2.7 Consultation time is limited in general practice, and sometimes only ten minutes are available to make a diagnosis and initiate treatment. Are there any salient questions to ask to help identify depression?

Don't be afraid to ask specific questions about the patient's mood, enjoyment and feelings about the future, using words appropriate to your interaction with the patient. It is helpful to ask about biological symptoms – specifically, sleep, early-morning waking, appetite, energy and weight-loss. Ask open-ended questions such as:

- How would you describe your mood? Are you miserable?
- Do you still enjoy things?
- Can you see any light at the end of the tunnel?

2.8 Are some people better at diagnosing and treating depression than others?

The most important thing is to have a high index of suspicion for the diagnosis of depression, since it is a common condition. Depression should always be considered in patients with non-specific somatic symptoms and in those with a 'fat file' (*see Box 2.5*). Elderly patients with recent memory loss may not be becoming demented but instead have depressive illnesses. Another common feature of depressive illness is the recent onset of self-medication with alcohol. Many patients suffer from more than one condition: depressive disorders may be present but go unnoticed in people who have other physical, or even psychiatric, disturbances. Screening questionnaires for patients and checklists for doctors are also helpful. The practice ancillary staff may have interesting insights to offer.

BOX 2.5 Cues for the recognition of depression

- Patient volunteers: 'I am depressed'
- Symptom(s) associated with depression
- Physical symptoms without physical cause
- Recurrent presentation of children by patient
- Doctor feels depressed by patient
- Doctor thinks patient is depressed
- Fat case-record
- Patients unduly troubled by symptoms
- Patients consulting without a change in clinical status
- Patients seemingly dissatisfied with their care

Guidelines on interviewing technique are given in *Box 2.6*.

2.9   Can you recommend any useful checklists for doctors dealing with a patient who may be depressed?

> A checklist of considerations when dealing with a patient who may be depressed is given in *Figure 2.1*.

2.10   What factors mitigate against the diagnosis and treatment of depression in general practice?

The most important factor mitigating against the diagnosis of depression in general practice is that the patient does not visit the doctor. Some 50% of patients will not go to their GP, in the belief that he or she is unlikely to be able to help, that they cannot be helped or that all the doctor will do is to prescribe pills. Those patients who do present may often give a history unrelated to an obvious mood disorder and talk about something apparently quite different; they may themselves not be aware of overt depression. It is therefore important to keep in mind the idea that mood problems or other emotional difficulties are common and may be a covert reason for attending the surgery.

The GP scores over the specialist by having a more longitudinal knowledge of the patient and his or her background, and it may be the repeated nature of the presentations rather than the specific clinical picture

---

BOX 2.6 Interviewing behaviour related to accuracy of diagnosis of depression

Early in interview
Establish good eye contact
Clarify the patient's presenting complaint
Use direct questions for physical complaints
Use open-to-closed questioning style

During interview
Use an empathetic style
Be sensitive to verbal and non-verbal cues
Avoid reading notes in front of the patient
Cope well with over-talkativeness
Do not concentrate on the patient's past history

Things to think about with a depressed patient

Name	Date	Date	Date
Ask about			
Physical complaints, including pain			
Fatigue/insomnia			
Loss of concentration			
Difficulty in making decisions			
Loss of interest or pleasure			
Low mood or sadness			
Abnormal self-reproach, pessimism			
Inability to feel			
Weeping, shame			
Loss of interest in normal pleasures			
Unable to cope			
Feeling hopeless/helpless			
Wishing to escape			
Ideas of self-harm or suicide			
Warning signs			
Substantial suicide risk			
Excitement, rapid speech, history of mania			
Heavy alcohol use			
Drug treatment			
Drug and dosage			
Side-effects			
Drug change			
Date drug started			
Date drug stopped			
Other options			
Counselling			
Relaxation or cognitive therapy			
Community psychiatric nurse			
Social worker			
Referral to psychiatrist			

▲

Fig. 2.1 Checklist of considerations when dealing with a patient who may be depressed.

that provide the clue to the diagnosis. However, the usual factors, such as lack of proper consultation time, may be a barrier. Another common problem is communication difficulties between doctor and patient in the areas of language, attitude and cultural divides. Either the doctor or the patient may not be attuned to talking about emotional matters.

2.11 When should a GP refer a depressed patient to a psychiatrist?

When there are difficulties in assessing the patient or making a proper diagnosis of the condition, and when patients have complex problems that need more than the straightforward assessment techniques available in the GP practice. Often patients have a *dual diagnosis*, with personality, drug and mood problems, possibly associated with psychotic illness. Such complex matters are probably best referred to a psychiatrist.

The obvious second group who should be referred consists of patients who have responded poorly to standard treatments – one or two courses of antidepressants given at full therapeutic doses have failed. A third group consists of those with complex management problems – especially those who are potentially suicidal. The GP needs to be aware of what the local psychiatric service can offer. Some offer assessments by competent and sensitive consultants who have a large array of therapeutic facilities and resources to hand. Other services that are more geared-up to dealing with 'the seriously mentally ill' may not be able to offer much in the way of treatment of less serious depressive illness – more the management of long-term chronic schizophrenics in the community. Under these circumstances patients do not necessarily do better if referred to a specialist and may never get beyond the screener of the Community Mental Health Team.

2.12 Sometimes physical illness is misdiagnosed as depression and vice versa – an example being chronic fatigue syndrome. Why is this, and how can we be sure of the right diagnosis?

The question is fundamental to the mind–body dichotomy issue and covers many important areas. One issue is the fear of making a wrong diagnosis – it does happen, when misdiagnosing a brain tumour as depression, for example. Tragically this has happened to many of us, and we never forget it. We all remember the rare occasions we have missed a serious treatable physical illness and thought of it as psychological, but we quite frequently miss treatable depressions or over-investigate patients for spurious organic conditions 'just to be on the safe side'. Many patients have mild somatoform disorders – a preoccupation with their physical health which brings them to their GP's attention more often than less preoccupied individuals. Sometimes physical abnormalities are found, but treating them does not necessarily cure the patient.

Chronic fatigue syndrome is an example where there may be a genuine fatigue state for which no obvious organic cause can be found, which may not be the consequence of a classic depressive illness. At this point one treats symptomatically both along supportive, behavioural and possibly even medical lines. The idea that chronic fatigue syndrome is a variant of ME, a viral illness affecting the brain and muscles for which there is no treatment, is not true or helpful to the patient. Being sure of the right diagnosis is really a matter of having clinical skills, looking back over the past history and taking the whole picture into account rather than pursuing obscure organic diagnoses.

 PATIENT QUESTIONS

2.13 What are the main symptoms of depression?

The fundamental symptoms are those of a low mood, unhappiness, anxiety, self-doubt, guilt and a feeling that life is not worth living. Other symptoms include a lack of enjoyment and a feeling of gloom. There are many individual symptoms of depression; each has a particular meaning for the patient. Some are more important to doctors than others. Some patients suffer the biological symptoms of depression, such as weight loss, loss of appetite, reduced interest in sex, poor sleep with early morning waking, and multiple vague aches and pains.

2.14 Will my employer have to know that I have depression?

That depends on whether you consent to your employer having access to medical information. Your GP may choose to make a non-committal diagnosis such as 'viral illness' or 'debility' on your sick note. Sometimes a white lie will suffice. If you have been off work for a long time, then your employer will probably want to know what is wrong and may refer you to an occupational physician, in which case the truth will out.

Many employees experience depression, and employers are usually very sympathetic once they know what the problem is, having encountered it many times before. If your employer discriminates against you by virtue of a mental illness you may have recourse in law. Before your employer is entitled to receive any information about you, you have to sign a form allowing your information to be accessed. You can always refuse to allow your employer access to the information. But this may have its own consequences.

2.15 Will having a diagnosis of depression affect my chances of getting life insurance or a mortgage?

The diagnosis of depression should not affect your chances of getting a mortgage, provided you have a reasonable means of repaying the loan.

Lenders don't usually look at your medical history these days, only at the value of the property and your ability to keep up the payments. Life insurance is a more complicated matter, especially if you have had previous episodes of attempted suicide. Your premiums may be loaded if your condition is severe. However, the practice of linking life insurance to a mortgage is less common these days than it used to be.

2.16   What should I do if I suspect someone I know well is depressed?

Encourage him or her to talk and allow time to listen to your friend's story in a non-judgemental way, so that there is no feeling of being abandoned, alone, hopeless and isolation. Encourage your friend to seek treatment, initially from a GP – GPs have considerable experience in such matters. Alternative sources of help include the church, social services, help lines and support groups – you will find some contact numbers in *Appendix 6*, or try Yellow Pages, your local newspaper or your local library.

Encourage your friend to keep active, to stay in work, if possible, to eat healthily, to drink alcohol only in moderation and to try not to let his or her symptoms gain the upper hand. Do not criticize your friend or say, 'Pull yourself together'. There is often a reluctance, out of embarrassment, to approach a friend who has a problem, but providing you go about it gently and sympathetically most people appreciate it – although you may have to choose the right moment to make your approach.

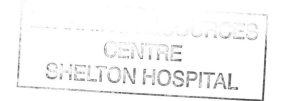

Different types of depression

MAJOR DEPRESSION

3.1   What is major depression?

The term 'major depression' comes from the DSM-IV diagnostic system. It is a condition characterized by either a depressed mood or a loss of interest or pleasure in most activities, lasting for a period of at least 2 weeks (*see Box 3.1*). This has to represent a deterioration from previous functioning. In addition there have to be four or more symptoms from the list given in the table below. The diagnosis does not hold if there is an organic cause, a bereavement reaction or other major mental illness or drug abuse. The condition has to cause clinically significant distress or impairment in social or occupational functioning.

3.2   How does major depression differ from minor depression?

Minor depression is similar to major depression but there are fewer symptoms – at least two but less than the five necessary for a diagnosis of major depression. The symptoms are of less severity and cause less impairment than in major depression.

Patients still have to be sad or have a loss of interest in nearly all activities to meet the diagnostic criteria. The condition blends into what could be regarded as sadness associated with everyday life, but, to qualify for a minor depression, the symptoms have to be present nearly every day and cause significant distress or impairment.

BOX 3.1 Summary of diagnostic criteria for major depression

- Depressed mood on most days and most of the time or an irritable mood
- Marked diminished interest or pleasure in all or most activities most of the day
- Significant weight loss or weight gain
- Insomnia or hypersomnia nearly every day
- Agitation or slowing down as observed by others
- Fatigue or loss of energy
- Feelings of worthlessness or guilt
- Impaired concentration or indecisiveness
- Recurrent thoughts of death or suicide

3.3 Is major depression necessarily 'more serious' than minor depression? By that I mean – is more morbidity and mortality associated with major depression?

Yes, almost by definition, major depression is more severe in terms of symptomatology and impact on the individual's functioning. Mortality is a separate issue but presumably it is a function of severity of depression. We know that severe depression is associated with a significant risk of suicide, a three- to four-fold increase in coronary events in those at risk, and a higher risk of premature death from many other conditions.

3.4 Is there any point in distinguishing between major and minor depression given that the treatment is essentially the same?

Yes, there is a greater imperative to treat major depression: first, because of the impact on the individual; and second, because of the type of treatment that is most likely to benefit the individual. We know that antidepressants tend to work better if the patient is more severely ill than if they have mild symptoms. Psychological therapies, and possibly St John's Wort, are more likely to benefit patients with minor depression. Antidepressant medication is of questionable benefit in milder depressions. Antidepressants are no better than placebo in patients with Hamilton depression scores of less than 13.

3.5 Is major depression more likely to recur than other types of depression?

Not necessarily; the type and severity of depression is not in itself an indicator of the prognosis. Minor depression can blur into 'sadness' or dysthymia (*see Q. 3.11 and Box 3.2*), which is more a response to the environment or a depressive outlook on life.

Factors influencing recurrence and relapse are multiple and not related to the severity of the illness, although the severity of the illness may influence decisions about prophylactic treatment.

3.6 Is major depression the same as psychotic depression or are psychotic features more likely to occur in a major depressive illness?

Major depressive episodes are further classified as mild, moderate or severe and with or without psychotic features and melancholia (*see Q. 3.7*).

When psychotic features are present there needs to be awareness that this may be a manifestation of a schizoaffective disorder, where there are not only depressive symptoms but also those of schizophrenia (*see Box 3.3*).

BOX 3.2 DSM-IV diagnostic criteria for dysthymic disorder

A. Depressed mood for most of the day, for more days than not, as indicated either by subjective account or observation by others, for at least 2 years. **Note:** In children and adolescents, mood can be irritable and duration must be at least 1 year

B. Presence, while depressed, of two (or more) of the following:
   (1) poor appetite or overeating
   (2) insomnia or hypersomnia
   (3) low energy or fatigue
   (4) low self-esteem
   (5) poor concentration or difficulty making decisions
   (6) feelings of hopelessness

C. During the 2-year period (1 year for children or adolescents) of the disturbance, the person has never been without the symptoms in criteria A and B for more than 2 months at a time

D. No major depressive episode has been present during the first 2 years of the disturbance (1 year for children and adolescents); i.e. the disturbance is not better accounted for by chronic major depressive disorder, or major depressive disorder, in partial remission
   Note: There may have been a previous major depressive episode provided there was a full remission (no significant signs or symptoms for 2 months) before development of the dysthymic disorder. In addition, after the initial 2 years (1 year in children or adolescents) of dysthymic disorder, there may be superimposed episodes of major depressive disorder, in which case both diagnoses may be given when the criteria are met for a major depressive episode

E. There has never been a manic episode, a mixed episode, or a hypomanic episode, and criteria have never been met for cyclothymic disorder

F. The disturbance does not occur exclusively during the course of a chronic psychotic disorder, such as schizophrenia or delusional disorder

G. The symptoms are not due to the direct physiological effects of a substance (e.g. a drug of abuse, a medication) or a general medical condition (e.g. hypothyroidism)

H. The symptoms cause clinically significant distress or impairment in social, occupational, or other important areas of functioning

Reprinted with permission from the Diagnostic and Statistical Manual of Mental Disorders, Text Revision, Copyright 2000. American Psychiatric Association.

BOX 3.3 DSM-IV diagnostic criteria for schizoaffective disorder

A. An uninterrupted period of illness during which, at some time, there is either a major depressive episode, a manic episode, or a mixed episode concurrent with symptoms that meet criterion A for schizophrenia [in DSM-IV]
   Note: The major depressive episode must include criterion A1: depressed mood [*see Box 2.3*]

B. During the same period of illness, there have been delusions or hallucinations for at least 2 weeks in the absence of prominent mood symptoms

C. Symptoms that meet criteria for a mood episode are present for a substantial portion of the total duration of the active and residual periods of the illness

D. The disturbance is not due to the direct physiological effects of a substance (e.g. a drug of abuse, a medication) or a general medical condition

Reprinted with permission from the Diagnostic and Statistical Manual of Mental Disorders, Text Revision, Copyright 2000. American Psychiatric Association.

3.7 What is melancholic depression?

This is a severe form of depression similar to what was called 'endogenous depression'. As well as the general features of major depression, there is a profound loss of interest in pleasure, a marked lack of reactivity to pleasurable experiences, the absence of a capability for pleasure, and a diurnal variation of mood. Psychomotor changes are present, and the individual looks depressed, not merely sad. Patients are less likely to have personality problems and/or precipitants as causes of the condition

MINOR DEPRESSION

3.8 What is minor depression?

This is a condition present for at least 2 weeks that involves a depressed or sad mood or loss of interest or pleasure in nearly all activities. In addition, at least two but less than five of the symptoms of major depression (*see Box 3.1*) are present. The condition must cause clinically significant distress or impairment in social, occupational or other important areas of functioning. Some individuals are able to function near normally, but this is accomplished with significantly increased effort. The condition can be difficult to distinguish from periods of normal sadness, but to make the diagnosis of minor depression the condition has to be present for most of the day for at least 2 weeks. Also if there is a clear precipitant then the diagnosis should be an adjustment disorder with depressed mood or a bereavement reaction. If the patient has previously had a major depressive illness then the symptoms should be seen as a residue of the major depression rather than as a separate entity.

3.9 How is it diagnosed?

At least two but less than five of the symptoms of major depression (*see Box 3.1*) must have been present for 2 weeks and represent a change from previous functioning, in the absence of any other major diagnosable mental illness.

3.10 Is minor depression more likely to be overlooked and therefore under-treated than more severe depression?

Yes, the boundary between minor depression and normal sadness may be blurred. The patient may be functioning near normally and the symptoms are not so prominent. Therefore many patients may not realize that they are depressed and may not present, and if they do present it is more difficult to recognize the condition. It is therefore under-recognized and under-treated, and more so than more-obvious depression.

3.11 Is minor depression the same as dysthymia, or are they separate entities?

Dysthymia is chronic low-grade depression, or a depressive personality. There is a low mood, present for most of the time, that has been present for at least 2 years. In addition, at least two of the symptoms given in *Box 3.4* must be present. There are fluctuations in the condition. Patients may also have low levels of interest, be self-critical or have low self-worth – these are qualities of the individual's personality, and they are often not reported unless specific questions are asked about them. The diagnosis can only be made in the absence of a major depression or other major mental illness.

BOX 3.4 Symptoms of dysthymia

A low mood and the presence of two or more of the following:
- poor appetite or overeating
- insomnia or hypersomnia
- low energy or fatigue
- low self-esteem
- poor concentration or difficulty in making decisions
- feelings of hopelessness

If someone with dysthymia then develops a major depression, the diagnosis changes to 'double depression', in which major depression is superimposed on dysthymia. Symptoms must cause clinically significant distress or impairment in social, occupational or academic functioning, or other important areas of functioning.

The main difference between minor depression and dysthymia is the chronicity of the latter. Dysthymia is an insidious, long-term condition and tends to be more chronic. It may overlap with chronic fatigue syndrome and ME or neurasthenia.

RECURRENT DEPRESSION

3.12 What are the criteria for recurrent depression?

The diagnostic criteria for recurrent depression are the same as for major depression, with the exception that there has been more than one episode (*see Box 3.5*). There are some problems in determining whether one episode has continued, albeit with fluctuations, or whether there are separate episodes. There should be a period of at least 2 months during which the criteria for an episode of major depression are not met. This is in contrast to recurrent brief depression, in which the symptoms of a major depression are present but the episodes last for more than 2 days but less than 2 weeks – typically, lasting 2–4 days. They occur at least once a month over a year, and are not associated with the menstrual cycle.

BOX 3.5 DSM-IV criteria for brief depressive disorder

A. Criteria, except for duration, are met for a major depressive episode
B. The depressive periods in criterion A last at least 2 days but less than 2 weeks
C. The depressive periods occur at least once a month for 12 consecutive months and are not associated with the menstrual cycle
D. The periods of depressed mood cause clinically significant distress or impairment in social, occupational, or other important areas of functioning
E. The symptoms are not due to the direct physiological effects of a substance (e.g. a drug of abuse, a medication) or a general medical condition (e.g. hypothyroidism)
F. There has never been a major depressive episode, and criteria are not met for a dysthymic disorder

---

Reprinted with permission from the Diagnostic and Statistical Manual of Mental Disorders, Text Revision, Copyright 2000. American Psychiatric Association.

3.13 Do people with recurrent depression feel well in between episodes of depression?

Usually patients do feel well between episodes. Some only make a partial recovery. There may be minor episodes between major episodes, and indeed there are many variations to the pattern of illnesses among different individuals (*see Fig. 3.1*).

3.14 What is the best treatment for recurrent depression?

There are many factors that need to be considered. The general view is that the treatment that makes the patient well is the treatment that is likely to keep the patient well. After an episode has been successfully treated, treatment should be continued for a period of 6 months before being tailed off to prevent a relapse, which would be the re-emergence of the original episode. A further relapse may not occur for many years – if ever – and so there may be no indication to treat prophylactically. Before embarking upon prophylactic treatment one has to weigh the risks and benefits of treatment against the risks of relapsing. If the illness has a lesser impact upon the individual, the therapeutic response has been good and hence the prognosis for treating a relapse is good, then there may be no need to treat

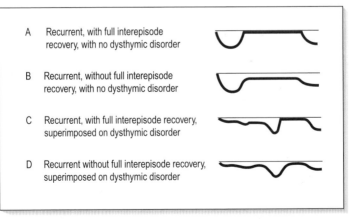

▲

Fig. 3.1 Different patterns of depression. (Reprinted with permission from the Diagnostic and Statistical Manual of Mental Disorders, Text Revision, Copyright 2000. American Psychiatric Association.)

prophylactically. If, on the other hand, the illness has a tendency to relapse frequently and have a major impact, for example resulting in severe symptoms or suicidal ideation, then strenuous efforts should be made to prevent further episodes by vigorous prophylactic treatment.

The indication to treat is also dependent on the therapeutic response, and also whether the side-effects are low. The indication for continued treatment may be reduced if the therapeutic response is poor and the side-effects severe. Whether to use an antidepressant or a mood stabilizer is a key question. The side-effects with the modern antidepressants would appear to be less than with mood stabilizers, and there is a respectable body of expertise being built up regarding long-term antidepressant medication. They are the correct treatment of first choice to prevent recurrence (a new episode) and probably to prevent relapse (the breaking through of suppressed symptoms in a current episode). In general, the side-effects of modern antidepressants are less than those of lithium, carbamazepine or sodium valproate. The reason for not using antidepressants is that they may promote swings into mania or rapid cycling (a small theoretical risk). Also if a patient is on full doses of antidepressants and then relapses, there is little additional treatment available if they become depressed on treatment. Conversely, lithium is cumbersome to administer, and regular blood tests are required.
It has its own side-effects and is potentially toxic, as well as causing thyroid problems and possible renal complications in a significant number of patients. Other mood stabilizers also have side-effect problems, and their use is less well established, although sodium valproate is gathering favour as a treatment of choice.

3.15 Should recurrent depression be managed in general practice in the same way as other chronic diseases – hypertension, for example? Should patients be seen regularly and kept on a maintenance dose of antidepressant?

The GP is ideally placed to treat depression because of the long-term relationship with the patient. The GP is able to supervise medication through repeat prescribing and review the patient regularly and should be available to intervene quickly should there be a change in the condition. Modern psychiatric practice is less suited to looking after individual patients long term when they are not ill. Continuity of care is critical. The patient should be reviewed by a psychiatrist at regular intervals depending on the nature of the condition – possibly once a year to maintain contact and to assess the need for continued maintenance therapy.

BIPOLAR DISORDER

3.16 What is bipolar disorder?

This is a condition sometimes referred to as manic-depressive illness. Variations in mood are universally experienced from time to time, as part of a natural cyclothymia. But bipolar disorder implies a greater severity of variation, constituting an illness. It is divided into bipolar 1, in which the predominant illness is one of recurrent manic episodes with associated depressive episodes, and bipolar 2, in which the predominant clinical picture is one of recurrent depressive episodes with mild, subclinical hypomanic ones. Patients are not only prone to recurrent episodes of depression, but when manic they exhibit features of a heightened mood with cheerfulness and euphoria. Irritability and hostility are common, as is overactive behaviour. There is racing of thought with rapid speech and writing. Patients have a flight of ideas with erratic changes of thought, resulting in thought disorder with increasingly tenuous connections between the thoughts. Punning, clang associations and rhyming are common. Manic patients usually feel very well and have little insight into their difficulties. Although a state of mania seems an attractive condition superficially, it can be very destructive since patients can in a few days spend vast amounts of money, commit serious sexual indiscretions and do profound damage to themselves professionally and to their relationships.

3.17 What are the diagnostic criteria for this disorder?

Patients must have had one episode of major depression and one episode of hypomania or mania with a period of relative normality in between. There are various subdivisions in this diagnostic category, depending upon whether the long-term clinical picture is predominantly one of manic symptoms, depressive symptoms or, occasionally, a mixture of the two occurring at the same time.

3.18 How common is it?

Bipolar disorders are less common than simple depressive illnesses. There seems to be a greater genetic loading than with unipolar patients. The incidence is more evenly distributed between men and women. The prevalence in community samples is in the order of 1%.

3.19 Is the manic phase of the disorder more difficult to treat than the depressed state?

Yes. Patients often have little insight into their problems. They feel well, see no reason to ask for help, and compliance with treatment is poor. In addition, patients are often quite resistant to the effects of treatment, which consists of either sedation or mood stabilization. Patients often need admission to hospital to prevent them from doing harm because of their behaviour. Patients rarely engage properly with treatment willingly.

3.20 How do you approach someone with bizarre health beliefs?

As with all issues, the first thing is to listen and take a history to try to understand which aspects of the health beliefs are bizarre and why and what needs to be done. Abnormal illness behaviour is a large and complex subject with a variety of manifestations ranging from malingering, where the patient is actively seeking gain through feigning illness, through to hypochondria where they fear illness in the absence of evidence (*see Box 3.6*). Some patients are frankly deluded as a manifestation of a psychotic illness. Others just have the culturally normal beliefs of herbalism, homeopathy and other alternative medical practices. The next stage is deciding to what degree your intervention is necessary. If for example the patient is potentially harming a sick child by denying it proper treatment, then your obligation to intervene is far higher than if they have very little wrong with them really and choose to pursue an alternative therapeutic line, rather than conventional treatment.

As with all complex belief problems, it is important to establish a therapeutic alliance with the patient allowing them time to put their point

---

> **BOX 3.6 Abnormal illness behaviours (in approximate decreasing order of conscious control)**
> - Munchausen's syndrome
> - Malingering
> - Hypochondria
> - Chronic pain syndrome
> - Somatization syndrome
> - Body dysmorphophobia
> - Hysteria
> - Hypochondriacal delusions
> - Somatic anxiety symptoms
> - Culture-specific beliefs
> - Depression

of view forwards so that you can understand what it is that they really want and through that relationship move forwards to a reasonably appropriate resolution of their difficulties. You have to decide to what degree you wish to disagree with the patient or at least put forward the conventional view in a clear and unambiguous manner so that they know what the situation is. One should be wary where patients have hypochondriacal delusions. This may be a manifestation of 'paraphrenia', or monosymptomatic hypochondriacal delusions, where people really have bizarre beliefs. For example they may think that a worm is eating up their insides or that they can smell gases coming through the floors. They appear to be otherwise mentally normal. It is a condition of old age and a variant of schizophrenia or severe depressive delusions and responds well to treatment providing it is recognized appropriately.

3.21 What drugs are used in the prophylaxis of bipolar disorder?

 Lithium is a drug of choice for the prophylaxis of bipolar disorder. If this fails, carbamazepine, neuroleptics or sodium valproate may be second- and third-line treatments, either alone or in combination (*see Table 3.1*). For unipolar depression the choice lies between antidepressants and lithium. Both are probably equally effective, and considerations of side-effects and cost and the need for monitoring of the plasma concentrations are

TABLE 3.1 Advantages and disadvantages of prophylactics for bipolar disorder

	Advantages	Disadvantages
Lithium	First-line treatment	Toxic in overdose and therapeutic use. Needs blood level monitoring
Carbamazepine	Established second-line treatment. May be better for some syndromes	Sedation. Rashes and other side-effects. May need blood level monitoring
Neuroleptics	Cheap. Effective in preventing mania. Depots good if compliance a problem	Risk of tardive dyskinesia. Unpleasant to take
Sodium valproate	Comparable efficacy to lithium, especially for mixed state and rapid cycling	Limited long-term data. Side-effects. Needs blood monitoring
Lamotrigine	Second-line treatment if others fail	Rashes and other side-effects
Olanzapine	Effective and tolerable	Expensive

important in governing choice. Lithium is gradually falling out of favour because of the need for blood tests and potential thyroid and other toxicity problems. Antidepressants appear to have fewer side-effects, but cost more. There is a risk that antidepressants may precipitate swings into mania, and for that reason they are best avoided if there is a bipolar element. Olanzapine appears as effective as neuroleptics and may be low on side-effects apart from causing weight gain. Sodium valproate is increasing in popularity. Since prophylaxis entails committing a patient to long-term treatment, this is probably best done after taking advice from a psychiatrist.

3.22 Was the name changed from manic-depressive psychosis because of the stigma attached to such a diagnosis?

The new names of these disorders probably resulted from the new classification systems of the ICD-10 and DSM-III, which were developed in the 1970s, before stigma became an issue. The naming is part of a more complex diagnostic system in which there are a range of subdivisions in the spectrum of bipolar disorders.

MIXED ANXIETY AND DEPRESSION

3.23 How often do these two conditions exist together or overlap?

Strong support for a distinction between depression and anxiety comes from work which was conducted many years ago, primarily on inpatients at the more severe end of the spectrum. This approach had the benefit of promoting more sophisticated research in the area but has not really added a great deal to the understanding of the basic processes. More recent work has shown that the stability of the diagnoses over time is not so good. Many patients can be diagnosed as having one condition on one occasion and having the other on another occasion. If anything, the diagnosis of depression is more stable than that of anxiety. Many patients fulfil criteria for both conditions at the same time (*see Box 3.7*). For example, in about a third of cases of major depression and anxiety there is an overlap, and two-thirds of cases overlap when comparing minor depression and anxiety disorders. In patients diagnosed with anxiety disorders, about half overlap with depression. Similarly, two-thirds of patients with agoraphobia and panic disorder could also be diagnosed as having major depression.

The conditions commonly coexist and are probably on the same spectrum of disorder (*see Fig. 3.2*). The distinction between them is often academic: sometimes anxiety is to the fore; at other times depression predominates. Most patients have symptoms of both conditions at any one time. For historical reasons depression is seen as the more important and acceptable diagnosis, and anxiety symptoms are often overlooked in the presence of a depressive disorder.

BOX 3.7   DSM-IV criteria for mixed anxiety-depressive disorder

A. Persistent or recurrent dysphoric mood lasting at least 1 month
B. The dysphoric mood is accompanied by at least 1 month of four (or more) of the following symptoms:
   (1) difficulty concentrating or mind going blank
   (2) sleep disturbance (difficulty falling or staying asleep, or restless, unsatisfying sleep)
   (3) fatigue or low energy
   (4) irritability
   (5) worry
   (6) being easily moved to tears
   (7) hypervigilance
   (8) anticipating the worst
   (9) hopelessness (pervasive pessimism about the future)
   (10) low self-esteem or feelings of worthlessness
C. The symptoms cause clinically significant distress or impairment in social, occupational, or other important areas of functioning
D. The symptoms are not due to the direct physiological effects of a substance (e.g. a drug of abuse, a medication) or a general medical condition

Reprinted with permission from the Diagnostic and Statistical Manual of Mental Disorders, Text Revision, Copyright 2000. American Psychiatric Association.

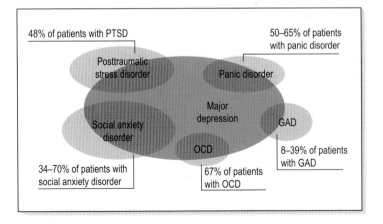

▲

Fig. 3.2 Overlap of mood and anxiety disorders. GAD, generalized anxiety disorder; OCD, obsessive compulsive disorder.

3.24 Is it important to distinguish between anxiety and depression when treating patients – particularly as several drugs are now licensed for the treatment of both conditions?

Depression used to be treated with antidepressants, while benzodiazepines and counselling were given to patients with anxiety disorders. This distinction no longer holds true, since the use of benzodiazepines for longer than a brief course of treatment is now discouraged. The two conditions have considerable overlap in their clinical features, and patients who present with depression at one time may well later present with anxiety symptoms and vice versa. Counselling and cognitive techniques are probably equally effective in both conditions, and antidepressants are also effective. MAOIs are particularly effective in anxiety states where depression is a minor component. Buspirone is the exception, appearing to be more effective in anxiety than depression at normal therapeutic doses, although its efficacy overall is in doubt. The current view would be to treat the most prominent symptoms by the most appropriate means. Many selective serotonin reuptake inhibitors (SSRIs) are now licensed to treat both depression and anxiety (*see Table 8.1*).

Since most treatments are probably effective for either condition and most patients seen in general practice have a mixed picture, the diagnostic category of mixed anxiety and depression in the ICD-10 and DSM-IV should be welcome. The debate will continue, however. It is often most useful simply to ask patients whether they are more depressed than anxious or vice versa.

From a prognostic point of view it appears that depression has a better outcome than anxiety in its more severe forms. It would appear that panic disorder may be a separate clinical entity, although the same therapeutic principles apply. In most cases in general practice the distinction between anxiety and depression is not very helpful, although it may have some validity in the more serious cases referred to psychiatrists.

3.25 What are the symptoms that discriminate between anxiety and depression?

The rating scales for anxiety and depression have many symptoms in common, such as sleep disturbance, anxiety, agitation and general somatic symptoms (*see Box 3.8*). Hypochondriasis is also present in both, as are intellectual and sexual problems. Key symptoms of depression are sadness, depressed mood, guilt and suicidal ideation with psychomotor retardation and general inability to enjoy pleasure. Features of high validity in diagnosing anxiety include fears, panic attacks, blushing, marked agoraphobia, derealization, and an age of onset under 35.

BOX 3.8 Symptoms of anxiety and depression

Symptoms that discriminate anxiety from depression

Anxiety
Fears
Panic attacks
Blushing
Marked agoraphobia
Derealization

Depression
Sadness
Depressed mood
Guilt
Suicidal ideation
Psychomotor retardation
Loss of pleasure

Symptoms that are common to anxiety and depression
Tension
Poor sleep
Anxiety
Agitation
Somatic complaints

3.26 Is there a tool that can help us distinguish anxiety from depression in general practice?

The Hospital Anxiety and Depression Rating Scale (*see Q. 4.33*) is simple and quick to use to distinguish anxiety from depression – it is filled out by the patient and scored by the doctor. But it is a screening test not a diagnostic one. It indicates whether further enquiry should be made. Out of a maximum score of 21 a score of 7 or less is non-case, 8 to 10 a doubtful case, and 11 or more a definite case. Both depression and anxiety are scored separately.

3.27 What is the best treatment for mixed anxiety and depression? Should benzodiazepines be used at all?

Antidepressants should be used for the treatment of depressive symptoms. If patients are distressed and anxious as well, then it is appropriate to treat them with benzodiazepines for 2–3 weeks while the antidepressants begin to have an effect, after which the benzodiazepine should be discontinued. Other alternatives are to prescribe a sedative antidepressant or a low-dose neuroleptic, but the important point is to build up full doses of antidepressants.

Many patients who are anxious are also intolerant to what would appear to be minor side-effects. These are unfortunately common when starting antidepressants, although they wear off as the therapeutic effect cuts in. Getting the patient over the initial 'hump' may be helped by starting on low doses of the antidepressant under cover of a benzodiazepine – as they say, 'start low, go slow'.

3.28 Is agitated depression the same as mixed anxiety and depression?

Some depressed patients express their anxiety symptoms in physical hyperactivity or agitation. This can range from mild restlessness to ceaseless movement, with hand wringing or skin picking. Pressure of speech is usually present, and the individual talks incessantly about the same topics. Patients may importune and fasten on doctors and nurses, demanding reassurance and help. There is difficulty in concentration, and patients cannot focus on the task in hand; they cannot stop thinking about the unpleasant things they do not wish to think about. Agitation is more common, and more marked, in depression occurring in middle life or older age.

SEASONAL AFFECTIVE DISORDER (SAD)

3.29 What is SAD?

The diagnosis is new, but the concept is old and was hypothesized by Hippocrates and by other observers since then. The cardinal features are recurrent mood cycles with depression usually starting around October / November and lifting in March or April, when there is often a mild hypomanic swing. The mood abnormality is not particularly severe, although it is sufficient to cause distress to the sufferer and those around him or her. About 2% of the population of northern Europe suffer badly, and maybe 10% suffer from minor SAD, or 'the winter blues'. The condition is found more in higher latitudes where seasons are more pronounced. It occurs more in young women than other groups, but children and adolescents may also be affected. One source of support is the SAD Association (*see Appendix 6*).

3.30 What are the symptoms of SAD?

Irritability is a common symptom of SAD, as is weight change – either weight loss, or, more commonly, significant weight gain during the winter that is lost during the summer. Sufferers experience work difficulties and problems with interpersonal relationships as well as problems with libido, concentration and energy and various physical symptoms such as aches and pains. In general, the symptoms of SAD are those of depression of moderate severity. Diagnostic features are summarized in *Box 3.9*.

3.31 What is the best treatment for SAD?

The specific treatment is with light therapy: daylight time is extended by the patient's sitting, for at least 2 hours every day in the morning, about 1 metre from a bank of fluorescent bulbs that emit either full-spectrum light (with a little ultraviolet) or 'cool white light' (without ultraviolet). An intensity of about 2400 lux is used – about the same as being outdoors on a sunny day. A treatment response should be noted within a week – there is a strong placebo effect. Treatment has to be maintained throughout the winter months for the effects to be maintained (or the patient has to move to a sunnier clime). Unfortunately, treatment with a light box is cumbersome, disruptive and requires a lot of time.. However, more-effective light delivery systems are evolving – *see* www.iguzzini.com and click on 'better light for a better life'. There is some evidence that fenfluramine (Ponderax) is effective in the treatment of SAD; antidepressants may also work, but strong evidence is lacking.

BOX 3.9 Diagnostic criteria for seasonal affective disorder

- Regular relationship between onset of depression and time of year
- Full remission or swing to mania at a particular time of year
- Two episodes of depression related to season in last 2 years and no other episodes of depression in that time
- Seasonal depressive episodes outnumber non-seasonal depression in the patient's lifetime

---

 PATIENT QUESTION

3.32 We all feel more cheerful when the sun shines – do we all suffer from SAD?

No. We all feel gloomy when the weather draws in and cheerful when the sun shines, but a depression has to be severe enough to be considered an illness. However, not all doctors accept that SAD is different from normal mood changes. Some mental problems are most common in the spring, whereas others are most frequent in the autumn. There is a strong overlap between normality and sadness. SAD is a syndrome clinically distinct from normality.

Depression in special groups

DEPRESSION IN CHILDREN

4.1   How common is depression in childhood?

Approximately 10% of 10-year-olds report symptoms of misery and unhappiness, but depressive syndromes occur in less than 2% of children and 4% of adolescents. Full-blown depressive illnesses occur in 0.15% of 10-year-olds and 1.5% of 14-year-olds. In child psychiatry outpatient units, up to 25% of children are depressed; and about half of inpatients have depressive disorders.

Depression is more common among boys than girls before puberty and more common among girls after puberty. Overall, however, it is rare before puberty and has a similar incidence to that in adults after puberty. Mania is also rare before puberty – presumably hormonal factors are important in the expression of the mood disorder.

4.2   What are the main causes of childhood depression?

Children generally respond to the problems in their environment. They become depressed as a result of loss – for example, the death of a parent or grandparent – or divorce. They may be subjected to bullying in school, or suffer from poor performance as a result of undiagnosed dyslexia, deafness or other learning impairments. If one parent is depressed, children can often develop depressive patterns of behaviour, either because of learned helplessness or possibly because of some genetic influence. Children may become depressed as a result of excessive responsibility in the family or, most importantly, because of sexual or physical abuse. Problems in the home, such as rows, financial difficulties or unemployment, also contribute to depression in children.

4.3   How can depression be diagnosed in children who might not be able to say exactly how they are feeling?

Many children are too young to realize that they feel depressed or to be able to describe their feelings. The important thing is to gather information from many different sources, including the child, the parents and community contacts such as school teachers. Many children present with depressive symptoms, but their parents are unaware of their significance; even so, a history should be taken from the parents. Children may manifest behavioural problems: poor performance at school, school avoidance, bed-wetting and nightmares. The children may also display feelings of loss, disappointment and sadness, aggressive behaviour, general disenchantment or a lack of caring. Depressed children lose interest in play and lack enjoyment in life, and this is probably the most important indication.

4.4 What symptoms should parents, teachers, health visitors and social workers look out for?

Any signs or symptoms that suggest distress or a change in behaviour should alert people to potential problems (see *Box 4.1*). Some children with depression have symptoms that are very similar to those of adults but with minor modifications accounted for by age, such as a lack of guilt and a limited vocabulary for describing feelings of sadness or despair. Many children, rather than expressing a depressed mood, present with unexplained abdominal pains, headaches, anorexia and enuresis as well as anxiety. On closer examination, a depressed mood may be reported. Often schoolwork will have a depressive content, and the child may lose interest and become disruptive or attention seeking. Depression may also present in association with emotional or conduct disorders or other childhood psychiatric syndromes.

Isolation, lack of energy, social withdrawal and, really, any behavioural change should alert the professional that things are not right. The precise symptoms are dependent on the cultural context, but the change in behaviour from normal is the critical issue.

4.5 How is depression treated in children?

Some children have clear depressive illnesses that are clinically indistinguishable from those described in adults. They may have a classic agitated depression and respond to antidepressant drugs, which may well be the treatment of choice. There is a larger group of depressed children whose problems are related to life difficulties, for whom the treatment is really dealing with and helping them come to terms with their problems. These often arise from within the peer group, or within the family, or are innate problems such as deafness. A third group of children present with antisocial or conduct disorders, school failure and drug abuse. These are symptoms secondary to depression, although the presentation is through bad

---

BOX 4.1 Symptoms suggestive of depression in children

- ◼ Abdominal pains
- ◼ Headache
- ◼ Anorexia
- ◼ Enuresis
- ◼ Anxiety
- ◼ Behavioural disturbance
- ◼ Conduct disorder

behaviour. Of course not all children with conduct disorders are depressed. The standard approach to assessing and treating depression in children is by using a multidisciplinary team of child and family psychiatrists as well as child psychologists, social workers and educationalists. Treatment is generally along psychosocial lines. There is increasing awareness of the benefits of antidepressants in children, although the evidence for the benefits of antidepressant treatment is not as strong as in adults.

4.6 Should all children with symptoms of depression be referred to a child or adolescent psychiatrist?

No, though much depends upon the circumstances, the competence and confidence of the GP's own healthcare team in dealing with such matters, the availability of local resources and the circumstances of the individual child, its family and social network. If the problem is relatively straightforward – the depression resulting from a bereavement, for example – then it would be sensible to adopt an expectant approach in the hope that the situation will resolve itself shortly. If matters are more complex, symptoms are severe and causing disruption in the child's emotional development or schooling or social networks, then early referral to a specialist is indicated – if only to set the process of treatment in motion before too much damage is done. Only a small proportion of depressed children are referred to a child psychiatrist or a paediatrician. They are most likely to be referred when there are behavioural disturbances as well.

Many children and families are reluctant to accept help. If there are concerns about the level of care the child receives at home or there is any suggestion of abuse, the matter should be referred to the childcare social work team so that enquiries can be made. The doctor should make a referral to the childcare team when problems are *suspected*, rather than waiting until they have been confirmed, since by the time they are confirmed it may be rather late to intervene. Referral to childcare social workers can open up a therapeutic avenue early on before the situation gets out of control.

On the one hand, managing depression in children is a complex and important issue, not only for the immediate benefit of the child but also to avoid a build-up of problems in the future and in adult life. The child is at a critical phase in its development, and damage done at this time will have long-lasting consequences. On the other hand, child psychiatric services are often overloaded, parents are reluctant to seek help, and the problems are often difficult to grapple with. A lot depends upon the severity of the problem, the availability of local resources and the family's attitude to help. If there is doubt, it may be worth making informal contact with the service to see what they can offer and what their recommendations are. There may be other agencies providing help, such as the school psychology service, visiting psychologists and, of course, the childcare social workers, if there appear to be domestic issues that are causing distress to the children. If the problem does not resolve quickly, then referral to the local service, not necessarily a psychiatric appointment, may well be appropriate.

4.7 What can be done to prevent depression in childhood?

Children with depression often have parents who suffer from psychiatric problems. Environmental factors are important, and the treatment of the parents and the family are also important in preventing depression in children. This treatment may often be along psychosocial lines. The first year or two of life is crucial in the emotional development of a child. A secure environment is a great protective factor against further emotional and depressive problems.

A stable home and school environment are important for maintaining mental health. The avoidance of bullying, peer pressure and excess stress on educational attainment are vitally important. Sadly, many of the factors causing depression are easily identifiable but harder to prevent. However, preventive measures include:

- a programme of positive mental health promotion involving liaison with local schools and youth centres;
- encouraging schools to be aware of the risks to children of bullying;
- the provision of counsellors in schools, as well as suitable out-of-school activities;
- help for parents in finding out-of-school activities for their children if they have to work;
- encouraging families to make 'quality time' available to the children, when the children are able to express themselves and are able to feel valued.

Above all, a secure home environment is essential to providing stability and the confidence that children need to develop normally and healthily.

4.8 What is the relationship between depression in children and adolescents and abuse of drugs, alcohol or solvents?

The causes of drug and alcohol abuse are, of course, multiple and complex. Cultural and social factors are very important, as is peer-group pressure and the availability of drugs and alcohol. Depressed and unhappy adolescents, as well as those who are socially excluded, are more likely to develop a drug or alcohol problem because they have less incentive than happy children not to do so. Once drug and alcohol addiction is established, the cycle of destruction, exclusion and deprivation continues. Happy children are more likely to find alternative ways of spending their time. Although many children will dabble and experiment with drugs and alcohol, those who are vulnerable by virtue of depression and unhappiness are more likely to develop dependency and a drug-abusing lifestyle. And some unfortunate children abuse stimulant drugs in order to self-medicate for their unhappiness. Then once drug addiction is established the condition feeds upon itself, resulting in depression and further drug abuse.

DEPRESSION IN ADOLESCENTS

4.9 What factors contribute to the development of depression in adolescents?

In many ways the same factors are at work that contribute to depression in children. Puberty, however, has a part to play in its cause, when the prevalence of depressive disorders rises to a level comparable to that in adults, presumably because of hormonal factors. Pressures at school relating to exams, career choices and possible unemployment are important, as are the pressures to succeed and conform and other peer pressures. The emergence of more-adult emotions and sexual feelings may be difficult to deal with. Sexual abuse is a powerful disturber of self-worth and an important possible factor to consider in a depressive adolescent. There comes a time during adolescent development when some decide that they will not succeed in normal adult endeavours and determine to adopt peer-group morals and social deviancy. It is important to note that adolescence is also a time when anorexia nervosa and schizophrenia begin to manifest themselves, and these conditions need to be borne in mind when adolescents present with what ostensibly appears to be excessive moodiness or other emotional complaints.

4.10 What specific questions can I ask to help me diagnose depression in teenagers?

A useful mnemonic device is HEADSSS (*see Box 4.2*).

BOX 4.2 The HEADSSS mnemonic for diagnosing depression in teenagers

Home – can you talk to your parents?
Education – ask for actual marks
Activities – ask about friends
Drugs – are they being abused?
Sex – is this a problem?
Suicide – consider the risk
Sleep – look for sleep disturbance

Changes in appetite, either increasing or decreasing, should be noted, as should the loss of interest in activities that are usually found enjoyable, such as sports and social activities. It is important to look for the signs of profound social withdrawal. Formal mental illness needs to be distinguished from the normal adolescent moodiness.

4.11 What can be done to prevent depression in this age group?

Essentially, avoid all the factors that can lead or predispose to depression, and stress the importance of a secure home environment, a good peer group and a stimulating and rich social life. Sadly, by the time disadvantaged or psychologically troubled children reach their teens, the damage has already been done. The first years of development are crucial to the creation of a sound sense of identity and personal self-worth in relation to the outside world.

4.12 What can be done to prevent the rising suicide rate in adolescents?

This is a difficult question. Suicide among adolescents remains at epidemic proportions. Despite an overall decrease in suicides in all ages by 15% between 1990 and 2000, and despite the Health of the Nations targets, the suicide rate in adolescents has remained the same, so the strategies that we employ have not been very effective.

The general principles remain: reducing access to lethal methods of self-harm since so many suicides are impulsive – physical means of limiting harm are of proven benefit; redesigning cells in Young Offender institutions, where so many episodes of self-harm occur; controlling the pack size of paracetamol and aspirin tablets – doing this has helped. Much of the work is along public health lines, since many disaffected teenagers avoid authority figures such as the GP. Those who are in touch with the services need more appropriate and targeted follow-up with appropriate empathetic therapists.

The identification of risk factors is important, and of course the greatest risk factor is a previous attempt. Those who complete suicide usually have a diagnosable mental or substance-abuse disorder, or both, and the majority have depressive illnesses. The best approach is to aim to reduce risk factors for depression – which often involve family interventions – early and to prevent damage being done in the early years of life. Much depression in adolescents is a function of social deprivation and exclusion.

Sadly by the time the issue becomes a medical problem, it is already too late and the damage has been done. *See also Chapter 12.*

4.13 Substance misuse and depression often seem to coexist in this age group. How should I respond?

Treating mood and emotional difficulties in people who are abusing drugs is difficult. It is important to control and stop the drug misuse early on, so that one can then make contact with the underlying individual and his or her emotional problems and make an assessment in the absence of intoxicating substances – drugs are often used as self-medication for underlying emotional problems or even depression, as well as self-harm and attention deficit hyperactivity disorder (ADHD). It is difficult to deal with these problems while drugs are still being taken. Once the drug use has been controlled then it is important to look at the underlying problems that result in drug abuse.

In general the treatment of drug abuse is of course not so much substance specific as dealing with the individual and his or her problems as a whole. The most important aspect of dealing with an adolescent who has a drug abuse problem is first to build a therapeutic alliance and, second, to start analysing what the particular problems are and how they can be dealt with. There is a danger that one focuses too much on simply the drug and not the whole picture.

ETHNIC MINORITIES

4.14 Why is depression expressed in different ways in different ethnic groups? Is it a different illness?

Depression and low mood are probably present in all ethnic groups and cultures, but their expression can differ markedly as a result of particular cultural norms. Western cultures are prone to introspection and awareness of mood. In some cultures daily commentaries on the state of mind are commonplace. However, other cultures rely less on the distinction between mind and body, and patients express themselves using physical terms, such as 'slowing down', or by somatization, with presentation to the doctor with aches and pains, and particularly pains in the heart. It would be simplistic to draw up a table of how different cultures express depression, but it is important for the GP to be aware of how cultural factors can affect the presentation of depression in different groups in their practice.

4.15 Some symptoms may be acceptable in one culture yet signify psychological illness in another. How can a GP differentiate the two when he or she may have little knowledge of the patient's cultural background and mother tongue?

Ideally, GPs should have some knowledge of the cultural beliefs and modes of expression of the community in which they work and be aware of any specific ethnic idiosyncrasies. If GPs are unfamiliar with these, then they should seek advice from family and friends of patients, and also from colleagues who are familiar with the cultural factors. The most important thing is to be open to the possibility that cultural factors can indeed affect the presentation of depression and other illness.

4.16 Is migration to another country a significant factor in depression?

Migration is a major life-event and can cause immense stresses that lead to depression. A great deal depends upon the circumstances of the migration, what has been left behind and what the future holds. An isolated immigrant who feels unwelcome in an alien culture is extremely likely to feel depressed, or at least unhappy, while people who have moved to a new life with their family and friends and are achieving their goals for life will be much less vulnerable.

4.17 How can doctors raise their awareness and diagnose depression in different ethnic groups?

The most important factor is an awareness that emotional illnesses in general can present differently in different cultural groups. To this end the GP should be open to diversity and be prepared to look beyond the obvious. It is important to be aware of the particular cultural idiosyncrasies. Doctors should attempt to learn about the cultures and social mores of the main ethnic groups in their area. They should try to define and interpret the terms used by their patients, for better shared understanding. Relevant literature should be available in the patient's own language. The doctor should not be judgemental but open and sensitive to the effects of not only the patient's presentation but also the doctor's own actions. They should be aware of potential concerns about confidentiality, and, for example, avoid asking children and family members to interpret if this is an issue. A patient's advocate may be sought early on if appropriate.

4.18 How can doctors in particular and the community at large help prevent mental health problems in ethnic minorities, and particularly in refugees?

The answer is really couched in social rather than medical terms. Refugees have often fled from appalling circumstances and may have suffered torture and witnessed the death of members of their family; there is often a substantial loss of status as well. The culture shock is massive, with linguistic problems, suspicion even among their own community and a whole host of difficulties. The way to deal with these problems is at a community level: to provide support, employment, housing and acceptance. GPs can often lobby on behalf of their clients, but the problem is not really medical. Early recognition and referral for any post-traumatic stress disorder may be indicated. Some specialist organizations deal with the mental health problems of specific refugee groups (*see Appendix 6*).

4.19 What is the role of somatization in the presentation of depressive illnesses in some ethnic minorities?

Many ethnic minorities are less attuned to expressing themselves in psychological terms. They are not used to introspection and expression of emotional anguish in words. Such people often present with physical complaints of either tiredness, weakness or pain. This is often of a non-specific nature, or an exaggeration of a genuine physical complaint.

DEPRESSION IN THE ELDERLY

4.20 Are there any statistics or studies to show how common a problem this is?

A quarter of all those over the age of 65 have some depressive symptoms. Most depressive illnesses in this group can be diagnosed as 'dysphoria of old age', related mainly to social isolation and adverse life-events, such as bereavement. In over half the over-65s, minor depression is associated with concomitant physical illness rather than primary depressive disorder.

More-serious depression is found in about 10–15% of this group, and about 5% have severe depression that warrants therapeutic intervention or referral to a specialist. The condition is common in this age group and quite treatable.

4.21 Do certain aspects of ageing such as loss of physical health, declining mental agility, bereavement and so on predispose to depression?

There is no single cause for depression. In most cases depression is multifactorial. These very real factors are, of course, important in the causation of depressive illnesses generally. As people grow older, the physical reserves to withstand external pressures become less strong. The biological reserves in the brain are also less robust, and the social reinforcers to prevent depression become less pronounced as bereavement and isolation increase. However, genetic factors become less important as a cause of depression with advancing age.

4.22 Is depression more common in elderly people who are in old people's homes or nursing homes than in those who maintain their independence and live in their own homes?

One-third of those in residential care have been shown to be depressed, so such elderly people are a high-risk group. One reason that people live in residential care is that they are more vulnerable to depression, either through social isolation or other vulnerability factors, such as failing health or mental functioning. People who live rich, independent lives are less likely to be depressed than those entering into institutions. Badly run institutions can be under-stimulating, promoting depression. Well-run institutions, for individuals who enjoy the kind of life they provide, can provide a very positive experience, adding structure and companionship to what would otherwise be isolation and loneliness. Much depends on the personality make-up of the individual and, of course, the institutional atmosphere.

4.23 Are there any tools to aid diagnosis of depression in the elderly?

The Geriatric Depression Rating Scale (GDS) is a helpful, brief, self-rating instrument for screening patients for depression (*see Appendix 2*). A score of more than 4 is above the threshold and warrants further enquiry. However, it is important to distinguish between depression and organic states; excluding dementia is also important. The Mini-Mental-State Examination (MMSE) is useful as a diagnostic tool for organic impairment and to distinguish this from depression. A detailed history and mental-state examination is probably the most important aspect of the assessment.

4.24 With older patients it can be difficult to discriminate between sadness and depression, especially when there is no biological shift. How do you do so?

There is a general view that old people should be depressed because of increasing age, social isolation and an associated failing health. The incidence of depression is of course far greater in the elderly than in younger people. It is so common that it is almost taken as normal. Depression should be treated whatever its cause and whether or not there is a biological shift. There are many treatments beyond antidepressants for such patients.

Patients should be encouraged to socialize, attend day care clubs and to keep active in a way appropriate to their needs. Community Psychiatric Nurses are in a good position to monitor the patient's daily situation with respect to their mood. If in doubt a simple mood rating form can be completed, such as the Hamilton Depression Rating Scale or the GDS. Physical problems and social isolation should be addressed and patients encouraged to participate in activities. If there remains a doubt about depressive problems an antidepressant should be tried. The situation should be monitored carefully over a period of a few weeks; if there is no obvious benefit from antidepressant treatment then it should be stopped, whereas if there is benefit then antidepressant treatment should be continued.

4.25 It can be very difficult to differentiate depression from dementia or CVA. Do you have any tips?

There are many similarities between dementia and depressive pseudo-dementia, a condition that mimics dementia (*see Q. 4.26*). The most obvious way to tell the two apart is by assessing the patient's memory. In depression, patients will simply say 'I don't know' if they cannot answer the question, whereas demented patients will either confabulate (make up appropriate answers), or perseverate (repeat the answer or the question several times). Depressed patients look sad; demented patients look vague. Demented patients also have visuospatial difficulties that can be detected by making them draw a clock face or other complex diagram. A score of less than 25 on a MMSE test is likely to be diagnostic of dementia.

If there is still some doubt after doing the careful assessment, it may well be worth a therapeutic trial of full doses of a non-toxic antidepressant for a period of a month to 6 weeks to see whether it produces a significant improvement. If the treatment does not demonstrate an obvious benefit, it should be stopped. It is probably better to over-treat someone who will not benefit rather than to under-treat someone who can be helped. Modern antidepressants are generally safe after a CVA, and ECT is also an appropriate treatment.

4.26 What is depressive pseudo-dementia?

A small proportion of retarded depressed patients present with pseudo-dementia. In this condition they have a conspicuous difficulty in concentrating and remembering. Careful clinical testing shows that there is no major defect in memory function. The condition can be distinguished from dementia by the history, which often shows a mood disturbance preceding other symptoms. Depressed patients are unwilling to answer questions during the mental-state examination, and this can be distinguished from the demented patients' failure of memory. In dementia, impairment is global, whereas depressed patients are likely to have partial defects. If in doubt, and this may not be unusual, a therapeutic trial of antidepressants should be given, and even ECT should be considered. It may produce miraculous results.

4.27 What is Cotard's syndrome?

This is a condition described by the French psychiatrist Cotard in 1882. The characteristic feature is an extreme nihilistic delusion. For example, some patients may complain that their bowels are being destroyed or that they will never pass faeces again. Others may assert they are penniless or without any prospect of having money again. Some may be convinced that their whole family has ceased to exist, or that they are empty and have no organs.

This is a severe depressive illness that should respond to antidepressant medications but may well require ECT.

4.28 Should the elderly receive the same range of treatment as younger patients, or should drugs and dosage be altered?

The treatment of the elderly is basically the same as in younger patients, with the normal provisos of caution. The elderly are more sensitive to the side-effects of drugs, and therefore the starting dose and possibly the therapeutic dose needs to be lower. The physical health of the elderly may lead to fewer functional reserves, and so antidepressants with cardiac or anticholinergic side-effects should be avoided. The elderly are likely to have treatments for concurrent illnesses, so antidepressants with drug interactions need to be prescribed with caution. They are also more sensitive to the effects of benzodiazepines and sleeping pills, which can cause confusion, and to the parkinsonian effects of antipsychotic drugs. All in all, care needs to be taken when prescribing for the elderly. Doses of medication need to be titrated up. But do not be afraid of giving the full adult dose providing there are no side-effects of note.

4.29 Insomnia is often a problem in the elderly. Should sleeping tablets be prescribed regularly to ensure a good night's sleep?

Sadly, insomnia increases in the elderly whether they are depressed or not. Some 20% of the elderly take sleeping pills, and, although this is generally frowned upon in the formal recommendations, GPs continue to prescribe sleeping pills and patients continue to request them. Providing the medication is prescribed cautiously, it may be a lesser evil than the distress of persistent insomnia. Prescribing long-acting sleeping tablets can result in confusion, disorientation, daytime drowsiness and falls as the drug levels rise and reach toxic proportions. The sleeping tablets may also mask depressive symptoms by giving some symptomatic relief but do not deal with the underlying problem. Regular prescribing should be discouraged, but in practice many patients become dependent and reliant upon their sleeping pills and are most reluctant to give them up since the medication offers them at least some comfort and symptomatic relief. On that basis it may be acceptable to continue prescribing. This is a view increasingly being voiced by GPs, if not by the regulatory bodies.

If a hypnotic is essential, the minimum effective dose should be used and the effects monitored carefully. Again, the more modern partial agonists at the benzodiazepine receptor are probably better than the classical full-agonist benzodiazepines (*see Table 4.1*).

There is no satisfactory answer to this complex clinical question since all treatments have their problems and complications.

TABLE 4.1 Alternative sleeping pills to benzodiazepines

Drug	Advantages	Disadvantages
Clomethiazole	Effective	Nasal congestion Interaction with alcohol
Sedative antidepressant	Treats not only insomnia but also underlying depression	Not effective hypnotic
Zopiclone	Effective hypnotic	Metallic taste in mouth Similar but lesser problems to benzodiazepines
Zolpidem	Short-acting hypnotic	Partial benzodiazepine agonist
Zalepon	Short-acting hypnotic	Partial benzodiazepine agonist
Barbiturates	Powerful	Toxic – AVOID
Chloral hydrate	Mild and effective	Dangerous when with alcohol

4.30 What can be done to prevent depression in this age group?

Old age is associated with changes in circumstances and with bereavements: often loss of the spouse, career and disposable income, sexual potency and so on. So it is not surprising that many elderly people feel depressed. The most important preventive measure is pre-retirement planning and counselling, especially in relation to financial matters and pensions, which cannot be begun too early. Alternatives to paid employment should be explored. Sexual dysfunction should be treated where appropriate. Incontinence can be particularly troublesome and may need treatment, possibly by surgery. The possibility of thyroid dysfunction as well as other significant medical problems should be considered. Mental and physical activity are important to health, and voluntary work and regular exercise are pathways to these. A good diet and a good social life also encourage well-being. From the medical point of view, you should consider HRT in women if appropriate. Bereavement counselling is also important. In essence an active, engaging life is protective.

DEPRESSION AND PHYSICAL ILLNESS

4.31 How common is depression in patients with longstanding physical illness or handicap?

As many as 20% of patients with longstanding physical illness may also suffer from significant depression. The depressive symptoms can be difficult to distinguish from those of the physical illness. The factors determining exactly which patients will develop depression are not clear and are not dependent upon any specific illness or patient variables. Taking the example of breast cancer, about a quarter of women suffer significant depression, anxiety and sexual dysfunction after mastectomy, and the risk is increased in those with poor marital relationships, unsupportive social networks, recent adverse life-events and previous psychiatric illness. Despite this, very few are referred to a psychiatrist. Many who experience psychological reactions respond well to brief interventions, such as one or two counselling sessions, or group interventions, including relaxation training and supportive psychotherapy. This approach shows beneficial effects on depression, anxiety and physical symptoms such as pain, as well as general well-being. Some work suggests that a 'fighting spirit' helps patients live longer, and adverse life-events may be associated with relapses. Some studies have shown that psychotherapy in patients with advanced breast cancer can prolong life. Nevertheless, the suggestion that the course of the cancer itself can be affected by the treatment of depression remains speculative.

4.32 Does depression affect the prognosis of serious disease?

Depression is a definite risk factor for coronary artery disease, increasing the risk of further coronary events by some three- to four-fold over that for non-depressed individuals after a coronary. Treating depression may improve that risk. In addition, depression is associated with an increased risk of other circulatory disorders, lung-disease-associated depression markedly worsens the quality of life, and depression may be associated with poor compliance with therapeutic regimes.

4.33 How can depression be diagnosed in patients who may be in pain and weak from illness?

Quite reasonably, many patients with serious physical illness are depressed. The treatment for this would be to treat the underlying physical disorder, as well as to offer substantial support and reassurance. It is important to ask patients how they feel and if they are low in spirits or depressed, and not just to think about the physical aspect of the disorder. Allowing patients to open up and share their feelings may reveal new insights. A nurse-specialist may have a better rapport with the patient and alert you to difficulties.

One screening instrument to detect whether clinically significant anxiety or depression is present is the Hospital Anxiety and Depression Scale (HADS), which is specifically designed to detect anxiety and depression in patients with physical disorders (*see Appendix 3*).

Taking a history from the patient about vulnerability to depression, guilt feelings, negative cognitions and lack of hope helps clarify the diagnosis. If the symptoms are present for more than a few weeks, then treating the depressive symptoms may be appropriate.

4.34 Many patients are already taking several drugs for their conditions, and it is rather daunting to consider adding an antidepressant. Do you have any advice to give?

Patients on polypharmacy may be taking as many as 10 or 20 different tablets throughout the day – and they may well be topping up with a few vitamin preparations. You ask whether it is worth adding one additional tablet that may prove to be of significant benefit. My view is that if the patient is already using a 'dosette' box, then one extra tablet is hardly likely to have a major impact on what the patient takes and may even have a good outcome and reduce the reliance upon other medication. The antidepressant should be given for a trial period only, and if there is not an obvious benefit after 3–4 weeks then it should be stopped. The patient (if he or she is capable) could be encouraged to monitor progress with a simple self-rating scale (*see Fig. 4.1*), either a homemade one or, possibly, a clinical depression rating scale or the Hamilton. This serves as a behavioural means of monitoring progress. It is important to have the patient on board in planning and executing the treatment.

The other issue is drug interactions. Most modern antidepressants have a very modest drug-interacting effect. Citalopram and its 'cleaner' analogue escitalopram are low on drug interactions and may be drugs of choice if polypharmacy is a problem. For drug interactions with MAOIs, see Chapter 8.

4.35 What other methods of treating depression are available to this group of patients?

Support, reassurance and explanation, together with therapeutic optimism, are probably as important as an antidepressant; counselling is a suitable adjunct. A good doctor–patient relationship is invaluable when it comes to encouraging activities to help to relieve social isolation. Sadly, elderly depressed patients do become isolated and reluctant to accept help or to go out, so this may be an uphill struggle.

4.36 What steps can be taken to reduce the incidence of depression in patients with physical illness and handicap?

Effective treatment of the underlying condition is, of course, critical, but dealing with the patient's fears of what the illness may lead to is also essential. Patients often think in catastrophic terms about the implications of their illness. They read stories about the worst possible outcome in magazines (and on the Internet), while serious physical illness undermines their feelings of worth in society and in the home. And their fears of further deterioration and death may well be true.

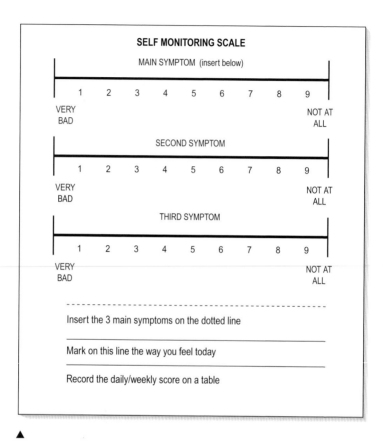

Fig. 4.1 Self-monitoring scale.

It is helpful to try to understand these issues and give positive reassurance. Ultimately we may not have all the answers for patients, but empathy, support and acknowledgement of their anxieties helps reduce the impact of depression. It is important to encourage family and friends not to abandon the patient, and a visit from the local clergyman may be appreciated. When it comes to longer-term handicaps, again a positive attitude with active rehabilitation and arranging for support services and user support groups to be available will at least minimize the impact. The idea that something is being done, as opposed to abandonment, is important.

4.37 What is a somatoform disorder?

Many patients are unduly preoccupied with physical symptoms which generally are not fully explained by underlying physical pathology. The patients suffer a great deal from their symptoms. They tend to be over investigated and frequently present to their doctor with various complaints. In the classical syndrome they have multiple complaints in various organ systems and this condition can be seen to evolve from childhood or teenage years. In some cases the condition is deeply ingrained in the personality. Other patients are just unduly preoccupied. The classic example of a mild somatization disorder is that some people will take a week off work with a cold and stay in bed whereas others will soldier on regardless. The idea is that the patient's response to their physical illness is highly dependent upon their emotional state. Many patients with somatization disorders have some depressive symptoms. The classic example would be a chronic pain disorder where the pain gives rise to dysfunction and disability, which gives rise to depression, which gives time for the patient to become preoccupied with their pain and disability, thus increasing the impact of the condition, and a vicious cycle is set up.

These patients are seen quite frequently in the GP surgery and use up large amounts of healthcare resources. They become very dependent upon their doctors. They are also a cause of great frustration to the treating doctor, who feels increasingly disempowered in his or her attempts to manage the patients successfully. Equally the patients are unhappy by virtue of their perception of chronic ill health for which little can apparently be done.

The treatment is ideally along psychological lines to help the patient understand the nature of their disability. The practical reality is that GPs need to be aware of this condition and manage it as effectively as they can.

4.38 How common are somatoform disorders?

A somatoform disorder appears to occur in about 1% of women and much less frequently in men. It is a chronic and fluctuating disorder that rarely disappears completely. It usually does not manifest itself fully until the age of 25 although it can be seen developing in adolescence. Diagnostic criteria are given in *Box 4.3*.

4.39 What is the difference between hypochondria and a somatoform disorder?

There are many aspects of 'abnormal illness behaviour' in which patients manifest varying attitudes to their perception of ill health (*see Box 4.4*). There is a spectrum of disorders ranging at one end from hysteria, where the patient for subconscious reasons develops a strong belief that they have some form of serious disability, for example a paralysis. At the other end of

---

BOX 4.3 DSM-IV diagnostic criteria for a somatoform disorder

A. One or more physical complaints (e.g. fatigue, loss of appetite, gastrointestinal or urinary complaints)
B. Either (1) or (2):
   (1) After appropriate investigation, the symptoms cannot be fully explained by known general medical condition or the direct effects of a substance (e.g. drug of abuse, a medication)
   (2) When there is a related general medical condition, the physical complaints or resulting social or occupational impairment is in excess of what would be expected from the history, physical examination, or laboratory findings
C. The symptoms cause clinically significant distress or impairment in social, occupational, or other important areas of functioning
D. The duration of the disturbance is at least 6 months
E. The disturbance is not better accounted for by another mental disorder (e.g., another somatoform disorder, sexual dysfunction, mood disorder, anxiety disorder, sleep disorder, or psychotic disorder)
F. The symptom is not intentionally produced or feigned (as in factitious disorder or malingering)

---

the spectrum is frank malingering, when patients pretend they have an illness in order to gain advantage – taking a day off work, for example, by maintaining they have a cold when they do not. Between these two extremes there is a whole spectrum of disorders. The patient's psychological make-up and mood influence these conditions and their presentation.

4.40 Should physical symptoms always be investigated extensively – even in the presence of a depressive illness?

It of course depends upon the nature of the physical symptom and what is an extensive investigation.

Depressed patients become ill, possibly more often than healthy patients. On that basis anything new or unexpected is worthy of investigation. If the symptom is non-specific and fits into the general pattern of depression then probably it is less worthy of investigation. This is again a matter of clinical judgement and depends on your knowledge of the patient. A difficult decision. (*See also Q. 2.12.*)

4.41 What is the relationship between depression and coronary heart disease and CVA?

Sadly depression is a high risk factor for both heart disease and stroke once the disease is established, and probably ranks just below hyperlipidaemia as

---

BOX 4.4 Different types of abnormal illness behaviour

Hysteria – The patient presents with physical signs which they genuinely believe to be true but which are in fact a manifestation of a psychological disturbance

Hypochondria – A fear that some minor symptoms are a sign of a serious illness

Somatization disorder – A preoccupation with multiple complaints for which no adequate physical basis can be found

Chronic pain syndrome – Complaints of subjective pain for which no adequate physical explanation can be found and for which psychological factors are seen as important in explaining the pain

Munchausen's syndrome – The patient deliberately feigns symptoms and signs in order to gain medical attention and possible hospital admission

Malingering – Patients constantly fabricate symptoms in order to gain material advantage such as compensation

Somatic anxiety – As a result of tension and anxiety, patients develop genuine symptoms – for example palpitations or breathlessness – which are a function of the psychiatric condition.

Psychosomatic complaints – Some conditions have a psychological component as well as a physical one. For example asthma may be made worse by the emotional state, or duodenal ulcers may be exacerbated by stress although the underlying pathology is clearly organic

---

an important risk factor. Depression is associated with all manner of increased mortality, partly as a direct effect of the illness and partly as a comorbid factor due to decreased activity, increased alcohol consumption, smoking and a reduced compliance with the treatment of the physical disorder. Treating the associated depression with psychological therapy or medication improves the functional recovery and possibly the prognosis.

4.42 Depression is often found in patients with other problems, including those with schizophrenia, alcoholism, drug dependency or epilepsy. How should it be treated?

Depression is comorbid with many other psychiatric conditions. Especially in schizophrenia, many patients suffer dysphoria and low mood as part of the symptom complex of the underlying illness. Many alcoholics drink because they are depressed or become depressed as a result of the social, psychological and physical problems resulting from their drinking. Similarly, drug dependency results in an unstable mood, often with depressive problems as the drug effects wear off, as well as the other problems associated with drug dependency. In epilepsy nearly 30% of patients have conspicuous psychological difficulties, and a depressed mood has been consistently found to be more common in people with epilepsy than in the general population. The most common causes of depression in epilepsy are adverse social circumstances. As always, treatment should be multifaceted, first dealing with the management of the underlying major pathology, dealing with social adversity and psychological problems resulting from the major illness and then dealing with the depression as best as possible. This may involve medication. Treating the symptoms of depression in people who abuse drugs and alcohol while they continue to poison their brains is a rather fruitless exercise. When treating patients with epilepsy, it is best to avoid epileptogenic antidepressants and also to be aware of low folate levels as a possible treatable cause of depression.

DEPRESSION IN WOMEN

4.43 Why is the incidence of depression higher in women than in men while the incidence of bipolar disorder is the same in both sexes?

Men and women suffer severe bipolar disorder equally, but, overall, depression appears to affect women about twice as much as men. This is not simply due to women reporting distress or seeking help more than men. It is known that depression is particularly high in women in socio-economic group 5 who live in isolated and deprived circumstances, bringing up children without adequate support. On the other hand, there is also a high incidence in socio-economic group 1. It has been suggested that middle-class women are particularly vulnerable to feelings of guilt, low self-esteem and depression, which they use to express their sense of personal failure. It appears that biologists, sociologists and psychologists can find suitable models that explain the statistics to support their own viewpoint. Bipolar disorder is predominantly a biologically determined condition with a strong genetic basis. Depression generally is much more environmentally, socially and psychologically determined.

4.44 What makes women more vulnerable to depression?

Vulnerability factors for depression in women include:

- having three or more children under 15 at home;
- not working outside the home;
- the lack of a supportive relationship with a husband;
- the loss of a mother as a result of death or separation before the age of 11.

Depressives experience more life-events, such as bereavement or separation, than normal controls in the 6 months prior to the onset of the disorder.[1] Thus the home environment and genetic and sex-linked inheritance may have a lesser role to play than social adversity. The role of female sex hormones may also be important. Their receptors are closely linked to neurotransmitter receptors, and mood changes can be closely linked to the menstrual cycle. Until recently, women still had limited independence, both financially and socially, and this resulted in their being trapped in unsatisfactory domestic situations.

4.45 What is the relationship between premenstrual tension and depression?

There is a considerable overlap between the symptoms of PMT and depression. At a biochemical level, brain 5HT systems appear to be blunted premenstrually, and antidepressants can relieve premenstrual symptoms (often when given for just a few days). Progestogens can also have an effect on the benzodiazepine receptor, and benzodiazepines can relieve PMT. On a psychological level, women with a tendency to depression are more likely to suffer from, or notice, the symptoms of PMT. In general if women are feeling happy and robust, it is easier to ignore or deal with the painful breasts, irritability and other aspects of the syndrome.

4.46 Is depression more common at the time of the menopause and, if so, is it relieved by HRT?

Although social and hormonal factors may have a part to play in involutional melancholia, depressive illnesses have a natural tendency to occur later in life. The concept of an involutional melancholia is no longer current, and it is probably coincidental that women complain of depression around the time of the menopause. The symptoms of the menopause should be treated and hormone replacement therapy (HRT) given as appropriate. Counselling may be offered. Whatever the cause of the depressive symptoms, it may be worth treating them with antidepressants if the symptoms warrant it.

HRT improves psychological well-being and relieves irritability, fatigue, anxiety and depression. It has been reported to cause depression, but this is uncommon. HRT by itself is not sufficient to treat depression in postmenopausal women, but may help improve general well-being in milder forms of depression.

DEPRESSION IN PREGNANCY

4.47 Is this usually a problem because women who are depressed may get pregnant like any other women, or do women sometimes develop depression in pregnancy?

Most women feel emotionally well during pregnancy. Anxiety and depression are most common during the first trimester of unwanted pregnancies, and during the third trimester there may be fears about the impending delivery or doubts about the normality of the fetus. Depression is more common in women with a history of previous psychiatric disorders and may be worse in those with medical problems associated with a pregnancy, such as diabetes. Although minor mood symptoms are common in pregnancy, serious psychiatric disorders are probably less common than in non-pregnant women. Some women with chronic depressions report some improvement during pregnancy. It is rare for depressive illnesses to develop de novo in pregnancy.

4.48 Are there any factors which predispose to the development of depression in pregnancy?

The most important predisposing factor is of course a pre-existing or previous depression. Unwanted pregnancies or pregnancy in those with relationship and social problems are more likely to result in depression, as are ambivalent feelings towards motherhood. In an unwanted pregnancy, fear of being unable to cope alone, the effect on a career and social ostracism are major causes for understandable but lesser depression. These problems usually resolve with time, although the long-term impact of an unwanted pregnancy may be substantial. Mothers generally adapt.

4.49 How is depression best treated – bearing in mind that most drugs are best avoided in pregnancy?

 As always, consider the benefits of treating the depression against the risks to the fetus; if the depression is severe or has a serious impact then treatment is justified, whereas if it is mild and medication does not help then it is probably not justified. Always treat with the lowest effective dose for the shortest period of time and review the situation regularly. If patients become pregnant while on effective treatment, it is probably best to leave them on the treatment lest they relapse if it is stopped. Although the true incidence of malformations with antidepressants is generally not known, the majority of fetal malformations are of unknown causation, and possibly 1–3% of all malformations will be caused by drugs (*see Table 4.2*). The maximum teratogenic potential occurs approximately 7–60 days after conception, although developmental problems may still occur in the second

TABLE 4.2 Relative risks and causation of fetal malformation in pregnancy	
Type	**Risk**
All malformations (including spontaneous abortions)	~ 20%
Minor malformations	10%
Major malformations detected by 5 years old	5%
Major malformations at birth	2.5%
Causation	**Frequency**
Genetic origin	20–25%
Unknown	65–70%
Drugs	1–3%

Source: Taylor D et al (eds) 2001 The Maudsley prescribing guidelines, 6th edn. Martin Dunitz, London, with permission from Taylor and Francis.

and third trimesters. The risk of fetal malformations may increase with polypharmacy. And of course pharmacokinetic changes occur during pregnancy, especially for lithium, and so this treatment needs to be monitored more carefully with a possible increase in dosage during pregnancy to maintain the therapeutic plasma concentration. Finally, withdrawal effects may occur in the newborn. The majority of pregnancies in patients with depression are unplanned, and so many mothers will be on antidepressants before they realize that they are pregnant.

4.50 Does the depression tend to lift when the baby is born or does it get worse and merge into postnatal depression?

Between a half and two-thirds of women will experience brief episodes of irritability and a labile mood known as the 'baby blues'. These reach their peak on the third or fourth day postpartum and settle. The blues are more common among those who are vulnerable to anxiety and depression.

Ten to fifteen percent of women develop depressive illnesses of moderate severity that begin after the first 2 weeks of the puerperium. Tiredness, irritability and anxiety are more prominent than depressed mood. Again, most patients recover after a few months. Depression during pregnancy is generally rare and does not disappear when the baby is born.

POSTNATAL DEPRESSION

4.51 What is postnatal depression?

This is a specific condition of a clinically significant depressive illness occurring in the mother within 4 weeks of delivery of the child. The clinical picture may not differ from that of a normal depressive illness. In some cases it may assume psychotic proportions. These conditions are often found in vulnerable mothers with difficulties in psychological adjustment to motherhood as well as the loss of sleep and hard work involved in the care of an infant. Stressful life-events are known to occur in mothers with postpartum depression. A previous history of psychiatric disorder at a young age, poor marital relationships and the absence of social support are also notable. It appears that the hormonal changes following childbirth are also blamed for the onset of postnatal depression. It would also appear that the condition merges into normal depressive illnesses in its causation and manifestation.

4.52 What is the incidence of postnatal depression?

Less severe depressive disorders occur in approximately 10–15% of mothers. The condition appears to have an insidious onset and a gradual increase in severity of depression over the first year postpartum, although in true postnatal depressions the condition should have manifested itself within a month of childbirth.

4.53 What are the symptoms of postnatal depression?

In general the symptoms of postnatal depression are not dissimilar in the mild form to those of depressive disorders generally (*see Box 4.5*). Many women feel especially guilty about having depressive feelings at a time when, they believe, they should be happy. They may be reluctant to discuss their negative feelings towards the child. There is sometimes a fear of harming the baby. This is a fear, not a likely event. Tiredness, irritability and anxiety are often more prominent than depression. There may be trouble falling asleep. Lack of affection, loss of libido and a lack of energy

---

BOX 4.5 Common features of postnatal depression

- Fluctuations in mood
- Lability in mood
- Preoccupation with infant well-being (ranging from over-concern to delusions)
- Mixed anxiety and depressive symptoms
- Some confusion
- Guilt
- Tiredness
- Irritability
- Fears of harming baby (unfounded)

can occur, as can appetite disturbances, anxiety and tension, self-blame and social avoidance.

In severe forms, puerperal psychosis may develop, which requires urgent psychiatric intervention.

4.54 What are post-baby blues (maternity blues), and how do they differ from true postnatal depression?

This is a normal phenomenon occurring in 50–80% of women, more commonly after the first baby. The symptoms (*Box 4.6*) reach a peak in the third or fourth day postpartum. They end by day 10. The patients often feel confused. Emotional lability occurs. The condition improves without specific treatment in a day or two, although it may be a forerunner of more-serious depressions. It would appear that hormonal changes after delivery are in some way involved in the causation of this condition, although there is no convincing evidence as to the exact cause.

4.55 What is idiopathic postnatal depression, and how does it differ from postnatal depression?

The answer by its very definition: idiopathic postnatal depression is of unknown causation. It is really another name for postnatal depression itself.

4.56 Does postnatal depression differ from depression?

The clinical picture of postnatal depression is in most cases not so very different from an ordinary depression. The symptoms include tearfulness and despondency, irritability, and a lack of affection. There is loss of libido, a lack of energy and anhedonia. There is sleep and appetite disturbance, anxiety, tension, guilt and self-blame. There is social avoidance, suicidal thinking, agoraphobia, anxiety and panic, poor concentration and restlessness. In addition to these non-specific symptoms, there may be specific fears relating to the baby. The mother may be frightened of being left alone with the baby and have fears or recurrent thoughts about harming

---

> **BOX 4.6 Characteristics of maternity blues**
> - Common condition – almost normal
> - Crying
> - Lability of mood (rapid alternations between euphoria and misery)
> - Confused feelings
> - Anxiety – tension and irritability
> - Mild hypochondriasis
> - Duration 3 hours to 10th day postpartum

the baby. It is important not to overreact to these, as they are not usually indicative of risk to the baby but an expression of the mother's anxiety that things may go wrong. The mother may feel exhausted and lethargic and unable to cope with chores. She may have difficulty concentrating, and some mothers exhibit obsessive tidiness around the house.

4.57 What is puerperal psychosis and how is it treated?

Puerperal psychosis is a rare condition, distinct from simple postnatal depression, in which mothers develop a psychotic illness in the weeks after childbirth. The treatment is very much the same as that of psychotic illness in general. The clinical picture is often 'mixed' with confusion and a marked mood abnormality present in 80%, as well as other psychotic symptoms. Patients may benefit from admission to a mother–baby unit where the baby can be safeguarded while the least damage is done to the mother–child relationship. The mother's parenting skills also can be assessed, and this may be important especially if there are wider childcare issues involved. Beyond that the treatment is along standard psychiatric lines. Lactation is usually suppressed so that the baby does not take in psychotropic drugs via the breast milk (but *see also Q. 4.62*). General nursing care is given. ECT is often seen as a treatment of choice because of its rapid onset of effect. The prognosis for acute puerperal psychosis is usually good. Once a woman has had a puerperal psychotic illness, she is more vulnerable to further breakdowns, especially after further childbirth, with a risk of approximately 25% after further pregnancies, and a 50% risk of further depressive illnesses overall.

4.58 What is the best method of screening for postnatal depression?

The best method of screening for postnatal depression is to have a good working relationship with the patient. There should be high index of suspicion for mood disorders in mothers who are not quite well in the puerperium, especially if there are few opportunities for the family and the mother to express their concerns over their condition.

If in doubt, administration of the Edinburgh Postnatal Depression Scale questionnaire can be helpful (*see Appendix 4*). Taking a proper context-sensitive history is also valuable.

4.59 Should all new mothers be screened for postnatal depression?

No, I think that would be taking matters too far, but GPs, health visitors and midwives should be aware of the potential risk of puerperal illness and to be sensitive to signs of depression and other emotions. If in doubt, it is appropriate to apply the Edinburgh Postnatal Depression Scale, or make more detailed specific enquiries about the mood state.

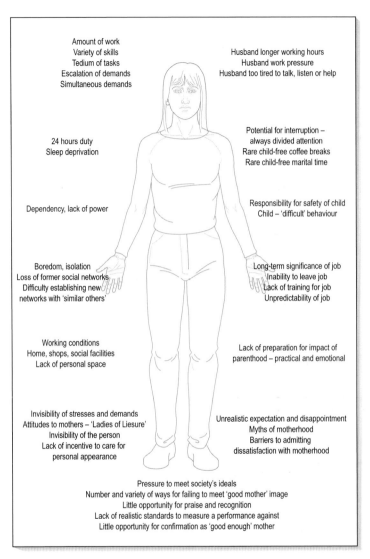

Amount of work
Variety of skills
Tedium of tasks
Escalation of demands
Simultaneous demands

Husband longer working hours
Husband work pressure
Husband too tired to talk, listen or help

Potential for interruption –
always divided attention
Rare child-free coffee breaks
Rare child-free marital time

24 hours duty
Sleep deprivation

Dependency, lack of power

Responsibility for safety of child
Child – 'difficult' behaviour

Boredom, isolation
Loss of former social networks
Difficulty establishing new
networks with 'similar others'

Long-term significance of job
Inability to leave job
Lack of training for job
Unpredictability of job

Working conditions
Home, shops, social facilities
Lack of personal space

Lack of preparation for impact of
parenthood – practical and emotional

Invisibility of stresses and demands
Attitudes to mothers – 'Ladies of Liesure'
Invisibility of the person
Lack of incentive to care for
personal appearance

Unrealistic expectation and disappointment
Myths of motherhood
Barriers to admitting
dissatisfaction with motherhood

Pressure to meet society's ideals
Number and variety of ways for failing to meet 'good mother' image
Little opportunity for praise and recognition
Lack of realistic standards to measure a performance against
Little opportunity for confirmation as 'good enough' mother

Fig. 4.2 Stresses of motherhood.

4.60 Do the stresses of motherhood predispose to depression?

Yes, quite obviously, stresses such as sleep deprivation, responsibility, isolation, loss of career, possible financial difficulties and lack of personal time are likely to be risk factors. Classically, having several young children and living in an unsupported environment predisposes highly to depression in motherhood (*see Fig. 4.2*). This is particularly so in vulnerable young women with unplanned pregnancies who come from unstable family backgrounds and who have unsupportive partners and families. For most people having a new child in the family is a joy, but for some it may be a great stressor, especially if there were problems in the pregnancy and birth, for example if the child is handicapped or born prematurely. Such socially caused depression tends not to present in the immediate puerperium but becomes manifest at times of personal crisis, when the long-term nature of the condition is recognized. The condition is common and often goes unrecognized or untreated. Most notably depression is common among those who have suffered it prior to the birth of the child and in whom raising one or more young children is an additional burden to an otherwise fragile equilibrium.

Being young, single and unsupported with many children is a high risk factor for developing depression.

Conversely, having a supportive partner or network, realistic expectations of new motherhood and a reasonable level of self-confidence protects against postnatal depression. In all matters, having support, structure and personal organization leads to a more controlled lifestyle, and this is protective against the more psychological or social aspects of depressive illnesses. Most depression after childbirth is caused by psychological and social factors. Having a supportive partner present during the birth and puerperium is another important protective factor.

4.61 Does a history of depression predispose a woman to postnatal depression?

Postnatal depression is a complex condition that is often really an extension of prenatal depression. Women who have been depressed prior to childbirth are often depressed afterwards. On other occasions it is a clinically distinct condition that may be a milder version of a puerperal psychosis. It must not be confused with 'post baby blues' (*Q. 4.54*). Having a young baby tends to be stressful in itself for a troubled young woman, especially if the mother is unprepared for childbirth and lacks a supportive social environment and partner.

4.62 What antidepressant drugs can safely be used to treat postnatal depression when the woman is breast-feeding?

 All psychotropics can be assumed to pass into breast milk, but usually the concentrations are relatively low and the exposure of the infant is slight.

Virtually no antidepressants can be detected in the blood of infants being breast fed by mothers on antidepressants. So there is really no appreciable risk. Antidepressants in breast-feeding should be avoided if the infant has impaired drug metabolism through renal or hepatic impairment or cardiac and neurological problems. Most mothers who will be taking antidepressants during breast-feeding will have been on them while pregnant, and the exposure to the infant will diminish after childbirth. If an antidepressant is to be given, it would be reasonable to avoid breast-feeding at a time when the drug reaches a peak plasma concentration (within 2–3 hours of taking the drug). This depends on the pharmacokinetics of the individual drug. As always, the lowest possible dose should be prescribed, polypharmacy is to be avoided and the infant should be monitored in case there are developmental problems. The choice of drug depends on whether mother was taking medication beforehand, in which case it would be best to leave her on the same treatment. As a basic principle tricyclics would appear to be relatively safe with the greatest long-term experience (imipramine or nortriptyline). The newer antidepressants would appear to be safe, but there is less safety data available. They have nevertheless been around now for over 10 years and subject to intense scrutiny and there do not appear to be any concerns over breast-feeding.

4.63 Is counselling better than antidepressants in the treatment of postnatal depression?

Simple support and counselling is a proven benefit in helping mothers combat symptoms and gain control of their lives. It is probably more acceptable to the mothers than medication, although antidepressants have been shown to be more effective than simple counselling. A lot depends on the severity of the condition and its duration. Counselling is probably better for the mild to moderate cases whereas antidepressants are more appropriate for the more severe and longstanding conditions. One concern is that whereas most postnatal depression recovers within 3–6 months, some 10% of mothers still have evidence of depression a year after delivery (a figure not dissimilar from that for depressions in general). It is therefore important to pick up those mothers who are in danger of becoming long-term depression sufferers and treating them vigorously, as the evidence is that the more vigorously and the earlier the treatment is instituted the better the prognosis. Again social support and 'sensible reassurance' is important. External help can be found through the numerous voluntary organizations (see under Postnatal depression in *Appendix 6*).

4.64 Do men ever experience postnatal depression?

Yes. Men do indeed suffer postnatal depression, for all the reasons that women do apart from the hormonal changes. Childbirth is an intensely emotional experience for men as well. They are often less well prepared for parenthood than women are. There will be pressures to support a family, plus sleeplessness and the need to make commitments. Having a new child is a major 'life-event'.

The Couvade syndrome, when the husband himself experiences some of the symptoms of pregnancy during the early months of pregnancy, is well recognized: most notably the symptoms of nausea and morning sickness and sometimes toothache. This complaint generally resolves after a few weeks.

4.65 Is there any evidence that postnatal depression affects the baby's emotional or physical development?

Postnatal depression may indeed adversely affect the mother–infant relationship, and the psychological development of the infant. It may lead to long-term bonding problems. The father may also experience distress. If the depression remains untreated, or becomes chronic, it can have profound effects upon the long-term family dynamics and welfare of the baby – not only his or her emotional but also physical development.

4.66 What can be done to prevent postnatal depression?

Hormonal treatment with oestrogens and progestogens in the immediate postpartum period may be intellectually appealing concepts, but they do not appear to prevent the onset of postnatal depression. The treatment remains experimental and carries the risk of thromboembolism. The recognition of risk factors in those vulnerable to depression, and the provision of support, both social and psychological, prior to the birth of the child are important. Most mothers who have postpartum depression may already have had depressive symptoms prior to or during pregnancy. The strategy of 'positive mental health promotion' should be instituted. This involves continuity of care, the development of social networks for mothers (often established at prenatal classes run by the National Childbirth Trust), postnatal support groups, mother and toddler groups and, if necessary, more-structured professional interventions to discuss parenting and the images of motherhood. If the social isolation is severe then referral to the child and family social work team before the birth of a baby may be invaluable in planning the postnatal support package. The GP and health visitor also have an important part to play in building a therapeutic relationship with the mother and observing for the early signs of the onset of depression.

Depression and sleep

5.1 Why is sleep so important, and what are the effects of sleep deprivation?

Sleep is a time when anabolic activity takes place in the body – growth, tissue restoration and rest. From the mental point of view, sleep relieves fatigue. Daytime mental activity is processed and filtered to that which can be discarded and that which can be stored. Natural sleep restores the individual to full vigour to enable him or her to face the next day with renewed energy and mental clarity. Sleep disorders are common problems in general practice. Twenty-five percent of the population are estimated to have occasional insomnia, while 10% have persistent problems with sleeping. Sleep deprivation results in a subjective feeling of tiredness, low energy, poor intellectual performance, irritability and moodiness, catnapping and poor psychomotor performance. Sleep deprivation has a small antidepressant effect in patients with severe depression.

5.2 How is sleep measured and quantified?

There are many variables to consider: the time taken before the onset of sleep, the duration of sleep, the subjective quality of sleep and the number and duration of nocturnal wakenings. Whether the individual wakes up early is important, as is the quality of awakening and feeling refreshed. *Figure 5.1* shows a simple rating scale. In addition it is possible to observe people sleeping either in a sleep laboratory or by doing simple nursing observations in their room at night. Sleep can also be measured at the patient's home using small recording devices. Patients will often claim they sleep badly whereas they are observed to be sleeping soundly. At this point there is the interesting quandary of whom does one believe: the patient who feels that sleep is unrefreshing and unsatisfactory or the observer who noticed no abnormality.

5.3 How is sleep affected in depression?

Sleep abnormalities are a very sensitive indicator of many forms of mental instability, and depression is certainly one. Characteristically, depressed patients have little trouble falling asleep, but then wake frequently during the night and suffer early morning wakening when they lie in bed ruminating on all the sins of the world. Some patients have low energy and sleep during the day, which impairs their sleeping during the night. Other patients have hypersomnia. Whatever the exact pattern, sleep disturbance is a sensitive indicator of the onset and resolution of depressive illnesses. Sleep is often one of the last symptoms to return to normal when a depressive illness is resolving. Initial insomnia at the beginning of the night is often a feature of anxiety. Typical sleep patterns in normal and depressed individuals are compared in *Figure 5.2*.

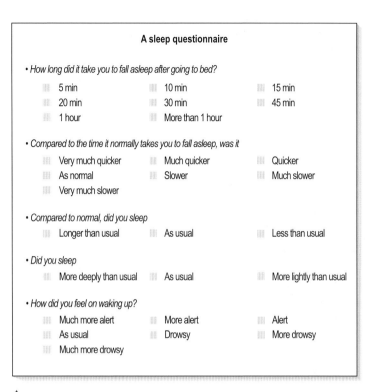

Fig. 5.1 Patient questionnaire for insomnia.

5.4 What is the mechanism of sleep disturbance in depression?

The precise mechanism is unknown but would appear to be intimately involved with the physiology of depression. In depression there is a delay in sleep latency, which is a consistent experimental finding. Sleep architecture is often broken. Cortisol does not suppress during the night as it does in non-depressed patients. The characteristic disturbance in the sleep pattern is in keeping with a biological rather than a psychological process in depression.

5.5 How should sleep disturbance be treated?

When sleep is disturbed as a result of depression, the most important thing is to treat the underlying disorder, namely the depressive illness. Treating the sleep disturbance by itself with sleeping pills is just masking the

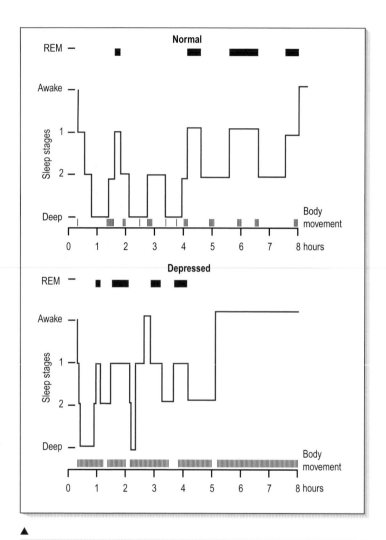

▲

Fig. 5.2 Typical sleep patterns in normal and depressed individuals.

symptom, which in the end is to the detriment of the patient. If sleep disturbance is prominent then consideration should be given to a sedative antidepressant – either a tricyclic such as dosulepin (dothiepin), or one of the more modern antidepressants such as mirtazapine which is quite highly sedative. Nefazodone had the particular property of inducing 'natural sleep', without being specifically sedative, but was withdrawn recently. If patients feel tired during the day, a slightly stimulating antidepressant such as fluoxetine might be considered.

5.6 Why is it that many patients request sedation because of poor sleep patterns yet show no other signs or symptoms?

As people grow older, their sleep patterns deteriorate and they develop insomnia. It is important to distinguish between sleep disorders for which there is no obvious cause and those in which there is – such as sleep apnoea, a depressive illness or a situational crisis. Providing people have had a refreshing sleep, even if it is brief, and if they have a stimulating lifestyle, they will have no problem with reduced sleep time. As always, it is important to establish a diagnosis before treating the problem. If indeed there is no serious underlying problem then, before issuing sleeping pills, there is a strong case for advocating 'sleep hygiene techniques' designed to help people to establish their own natural sleeping rhythms (*see Box 5.1*).

5.7 Is there ever a place for prescribing sleeping tablets in depression?

A small dose of hypnotic can be given for a few days in order to get symptomatic control early, and the hypnotic can then be withdrawn as the antidepressant effect begins to kick in while the dose is being titrated up. The danger is that patients will find the sleeping tablets so effective that they

---

BOX 5.1 Sleep hygiene techniques

- Self-monitoring
- Regular bedtime and rising
- Sleep only as much as needed
- No daytime naps
- Regular exercise
- No alcohol or caffeine late in the day
- If you cannot sleep, do not lie in bed and brood – get up and do something
- Practise progressive muscular relaxation
- Avoid excessive noise and heat in the bedroom
- Occasional sleeping pills are OK
- Try using a relaxation/sleep self-help tape

are reluctant to give them up even when they feel better, because sleep disturbance is often one of the last symptoms to resolve in a treated depression.

5.8 Why should patients become addicted to or dependent on sleeping pills but not become dependent on antidepressants? Do they become dependent on the 'feel good factor' of sleeping better and feeling less tired or is it a chemical phenomenon?

Sleeping tablets tend to work pretty immediately and reliably and give a reasonable quality of sleep in most patients. Their pharmacological mechanism is very different from that of antidepressants. Antidepressants take time to work, and, even when they have relieved depression, sleep may take several weeks and months to revert to normal. Patients become anxious at the thought of not sleeping.

Secondly, if patients become dependent on sleeping tablets but do not take a regular night-time dose, then they develop rebound insomnia and experience worse sleep if they do not take their medication. Many patients, especially the elderly, become used to sleeping relatively well with a sleeping tablet and cope badly with long hours of wakefulness.

Characteristics of an ideal hypnotic are listed in *Box 5.2*.

5.9 Years ago doctors welcomed the arrival of the benzodiazepines as they were thought to be less habit forming than barbiturates. What went wrong?

Benzodiazepines are not necessarily less habit forming than barbiturates but safer. The lethal dose of a barbiturate was not much greater than that of a therapeutic dose, and many patients died as a result of barbiturate overdoses, whereas it is almost impossible to die by benzodiazepine overdose alone. Over the years we have become quite rightly concerned about safety, and lesser levels of side-effects are now unacceptable when in the past larger risks were acceptable. The issue of dependency as opposed to

---

BOX 5.2 Characteristics of the ideal hypnotic
- Rapidly, pleasantly, reliably induces sleep
- Normal sleep physiology
- Wake refreshed
- No hangover
- Effective from first night
- Effects last for several nights
- No rebound insomnia on stopping

toxicity has only become an issue in the last twenty years. We all know that in medicine when you cure one problem, you immediately discover another one that needs addressing.

5.10 Are benzodiazepines as bad as they are now portrayed, and is it such a terrible thing that an elderly person might need 5 mg of nitrazepam or 10 mg of temazepam to help them sleep throughout the night?

Although daytime anxiolytics are prescribed much less than they used to be, hypnotics – benzodiazepines, and also the more modern sleeping pills such as zopiclone, zolpidem and zaleplon – are prescribed as much as they always have been. There were approximately ten and a half million prescriptions for sleeping pills issued in the year 2002 in England, and this figure has been relatively constant over the last twenty years. Most sleeping pills are taken by the elderly. This may be against the general guidelines published by learned bodies, but there is an emerging view that the latter may be missing the point, that GPs in the front line are responding to their patient's needs and that their patients are happy for that. The treatment guidelines are generally coming round to the view that long-term consumption of sleeping pills in the elderly may not be as terrible a thing as had previously been considered.

 PATIENT QUESTION

5.11 I have trouble sleeping but feel well otherwise. Can I have a prescription for sleeping tablets?

Before we take that step, it is advisable that you try some simple things to help you sleep. This includes taking warm baths, drinking a malted drink, taking regular exercise in the evening but not just before bed, and developing regularity of habits. Avoid daytime naps, caffeine and excess alcohol. You may wish to try preparations bought over-the-counter from a chemist; these are for the most part antihistamines.

Depression and food

6

6.1 Loss of appetite is a symptom of depression. Is there a neuro-biochemical reason for this?

The relationship between food and depression is complicated and not fully understood. Some people eat for comfort, whereas severely depressed people may not even manage to get out of bed to eat at all. Depression is common amongst patients with eating disorders, and the drugs used to treat depression may themselves affect appetite and satiety.

Appetite control is governed by a balance between 5HT and dopamine receptors in the hypothalamus. These neurotransmitters are of course intimately involved in the regulation of mood, and so it comes as no surprise that a reduction in appetite occurs in conditions where 5HT deficiency is postulated. Other forms of depression are associated with noradrenergic deficiency, and there the suggestion is that people, especially young women, tend to comfort eat. Where dopamine abnormalities are implicated, such as in schizophrenia, changes in appetite occur as well. Most notably drugs such as amphetamines and cocaine that boost dopamine and noradrenergic systems act as appetite suppressants, and antipsychotic drugs that block dopamine can induce voracious appetites and weight gain. Fenfluramine, an appetite suppressant, increases serotonin release (especially of $5HT_2$), and the classic SSRIs tend to reduce appetite. Mirtazapine, an antidepressant with complex actions on $5HT_2$ receptors, has quite a stimulating action on appetite. There is certainly a neuro-biochemical factor in appetite control, but the precise mechanisms are of course complex and unclear.

6.2 What is the relationship between folic acid and depression?

Very low levels of folic acid can cause all manner of neuropsychiatric problems including of course neuronal degeneration. There is some evidence that adding folic acid to treatment with antidepressants or any other psychiatric drug treatment can improve the therapeutic response to some degree.

6.3 Which drugs cause an increase in appetite, and can this be a problem?

The classic drugs that increase appetite are the antipsychotics which block dopamine. Olanzapine appears to be particularly potent at increasing weight although other antipsychotics can make some unfortunate individuals eat voraciously. Weight gain is one of the commonest and most distressing side-effects of antipsychotic treatment. Mirtazapine also is notorious for causing weight gain, but many other antidepressants have a lesser effect on weight gain. The effect is not uniform since some people gain weight and others lose weight while taking antidepressants.

Other drugs especially hormonal preparations such as oral contraceptives and HRT can have an effect on weight. Steroids are renowned for this, and hormones of course have a profound effect in modulating neurotransmission.

6.4 What foods are not allowed during treatment with MAOIs?

 Foods containing tyramine, which are specifically products of fermented protein, should not be eaten while on MAOI treatment. The classics are cheese, yeast extracts, matured meat, such as hung game, middle-European sausages and offal and, classically, rich red wines such as Chianti.

The list is long and exhaustive (*see Q. 8.36*). It is really a function not only of the food substance but of the amount and rate at which it is consumed. A small amount of tyramine can easily be tolerated, but a large bolus can be harmful. Phenylethyl alanine may also cause problems, especially headaches. This is found in chocolate.

6.5 What might happen if a patient on an MAOI lapsed and drank some Chianti or ate cheese?

 Probably drinking Chianti, unless a large amount were taken, would not be a major problem, but eating cheese in substantial amounts (cauliflower cheese or macaroni cheese are the classic culprits) would result in headache, flushing and a feeling of unwellness. Blood pressure would be raised, there might be palpitations, and in extreme cases the patient might suffer the effects of malignant hypertension and possibly a cerebral bleed or malignant hyperpyrexia or the 'serotonin syndrome' (*see Q. 8.16*).

6.6 What proportion of patients who suffer from anorexia nervosa or bulimia have coexisting depression?

Eating disorders and mood are intimately interrelated. People with eating disorders often have underlying feelings of inadequacy and dysphoria. They rarely have classic depressive illnesses and often feel quite cheerful, especially when they control their body weight. When their body weight is out of control they feel despairing but not necessarily clinically depressed. Anorexic patients often have high energy. They often lack insight.

6.7 Why is fluoxetine effective in the treatment of bulimia?

Craving as is found in substance abuse bears some similarity to food craving in bulimia. Serotonin is involved in this mechanism. Serotonin (5HT) also regulates a feeling of satiation, and SSRIs are associated with a loss of appetite especially at the higher doses and particularly in the case of fluoxetine. Abnormalities of the serotonin system are noted especially in obese subjects, and vomiting can alter the balance of serotonin and other neurotransmitters in the brain. Carbohydrates also increase brain uptake of tryptophan. The mechanism is not fully understood but there are many pointers, and the evidence is that high doses of SSRIs are significantly superior to placebo in decreasing binge eating and vomiting in the treatment of bulimia.

6.8 What is the role of omega-3 fatty acids in the treatment of depression?

Treatment with omega-3 fatty acids has been shown to enhance the antidepressant effect of antidepressants by a significant degree. This involves giving 1-g capsules of 96% fish-oil-derived ethyl eicosapentaenoic acid (E-EPA) as an adjunct to the pharmaceutical medication. Similar results have been found for treatment of other psychiatric conditions, including psychosis and dyslexia.

6.9 Has any work been done to estimate what proportion of people with gross obesity suffer from depression?

Grossly obese patients have low energy and feelings of inadequacy. I think this is mainly socially generated rather than resulting from biochemical mechanisms. Again classical depression is probably not much commoner among obese people than in those of normal weight.

6.10 There is a new anti-obesity drug in preparation (SNAP-7941) that is said to have antidepressant properties similar to those of fluoxetine and anti-anxiety effects similar to those of chlordiazepoxide and buspirone. Do you have any comments to make about it?

We have seen that modulation of the serotonin system has demonstrated antidepressant, anti-anxiety and anti-appetite effects. The targeted therapeutic area may be as much a function of marketing as pharmacology.

6.11 Why doesn't venlafaxine affect appetite and sibutramine act as an antidepressant?

CASE STUDY 6.1

An overweight patient (BMI 34) had been treated with orlistat with little success and desperately wanted to lose weight. Her GP wanted to treat her with sibutramine but was unable to do so because the patient was already taking 150 mg of venlafaxine, which is also a 5HT/noradrenaline reuptake inhibitor. Both GP and patient wondered why two drugs of the same class should have different actions – one as an antidepressant and the other as a weight-reducing treatment

The basic difference between sibutramine and venlafaxine is in the ratio of serotonin and noradrenergic reuptake inhibition. Sibutramine causes approximately equal proportions of serotonin and noradrenaline reuptake inhibition whereas venlafaxine predominantly promotes serotonin reuptake inhibition. This is thought to be the reason for the difference in the therapeutic effects of these two medications. Increased action on the noradrenergic receptor may underlie the mechanism of satiation. Sibutramine is not an appetite suppressant but helps patients feel satisfied with smaller portions of food, so they eat less. Although sibutramine has shown potential antidepressant activity in animal studies, there is no clinical evidence of its use in depression. It may well be an antidepressant. Clearly, defining psychoactive agents purely in terms of the reuptake inhibition potencies is insufficient to describe their total mechanism of action, although product development and marketing strategies also come into play when defining exactly what a drug is licensed for.

 PATIENT QUESTIONS

6.12 What will happen to me if I eat cheese when I am taking my (MAOI) tablets?

If you eat a lot of cheese or the other food or drink on the list I am giving you, you will probably get a headache and feel flushed and unwell. Your blood pressure will rise and you may experience palpitations. You may also be at risk of much more serious side-effects – 'serotonin syndrome', severe high blood pressure or bleeding in the brain.

6.13 Can we make ourselves happier by eating? Are there substances in some foods that act as antidepressants?

The food ingredient whose absence from a diet is most clearly implicated in depression is called tryptophan. It is related to the brain chemical serotonin, which is important in mood control. When volunteers have been fed food which is low in tryptophan they have become acutely depressed, and feeding vast amounts of tryptophan, in the form of L-tryptophan, acts as a weak antidepressant. More importantly, however, you should try to avoid comfort eating; this will have little more than a short-term mood-enhancing effect but may make you feel worse in the long term as a result of weight gain.

Depression and sex

7

7.1 What is the link between depression and sex?

Sexual problems and depression are both common problems in general practice and psychiatry. One study in primary care has shown that 20% of women describe difficulty in becoming aroused, and 7% are anorgasmic. Seven percent of men described transient erectile problems, while 20% reported premature ejaculation.[1] In an outpatient setting sexual problems were found in 36% of patients with affective disorder.[2] This is hardly surprising since dopamine facilitates sexual activity and noradrenaline has central actions which increase arousal and peripheral effects which may impair sexual performance. Serotonin inhibits sexual function via $5HT_2$ pathways.

Sexual problems and depression may occur together or as a consequence of each other. Thus depression and its treatment may lead to sexual problems, while repeated sexual problems may be a cause of depression. It is important to take a good history to try and find out which came first.

Sexual problems are usually categorized as:

- disorders of desire – where there is lack of or loss of libido, sometimes leading to the avoidance of sex altogether
- disorders of arousal – in which the normal genital sexual response of vaginal lubrication in women and penile erection in men does not occur or occurs insufficiently
- disorders of orgasm – in which men fail to ejaculate and women do not climax and have an orgasm.

There are also disorders of sexual pain (vaginismus or dyspareunia) and other unspecified sexual disorders, though these are not usually associated with depression and its treatment.

7.2 Why should depression affect sexual activity and enjoyment?

Depression affects sexual enjoyment and drive, and is one of the most sensitive early indices of impairment is in this area. Relationships become affected, resulting in irritability and communication difficulties. Patients withdraw from their partners. It is not surprising that a low mood affects the ability to enjoy sex. Paradoxically, some individuals find comfort in sexual activity, using it as an antidepressant to offer a demonstration of continued love for their partner, and find continued sexual activity important as a validation of themselves.

7.3 How important is it to take a proper sexual history when treating depression?

It may not be the most important question to ask, but enquiries need to be made to make a proper assessment. Most of all, sexual abuse in childhood or in ongoing relationships may be an important causative factor relating to personality vulnerabilities predisposing to depression. Patients will often avoid talking about sexual abuse in childhood, and even deny it until they feel comfortable and familiar with the doctor. The issue needs sensitive handling and may not emerge until the second or third interview. More-recent sexual problems may give a clue to current relationship difficulties, marital infidelity, morbid jealousy or ongoing psychological difficulties. It may also be an index of the severity of the current depression. It may well be coincidental to the patient and not important at all. Finally it is important to warn the patient that taking antidepressants may result in a worsening of sexual performance, usually by delaying orgasm. If patients are not warned, this can cause further concerns. Usually when warned they are prepared to tolerate this particular problem if there is a prospect that they will become well again otherwise. Drugs and alcohol need to be asked about because they can of course impair sexual performance as well.

7.4 How can I distinguish between pre-existing sexual problems and those caused by depression and its treatment?

As always, a detailed history is important. Once the question is broached with patients they are often pleased to talk about it openly and frankly. There are three areas to enquire about:

- whether the patient had sexual problems prior to the onset of the depressive illness
- the problems during the depression
- the problems resulting from the treatment.

You can gauge a level of concern in the patient and decide whether this should become a focus for further investigation. Psychosexual counselling may be appropriate, but is best left until the depressive illness is treated appropriately. Patients often welcome the opportunity of discussing their sexual problems and the realization that they are not alone or unusual. Two out of three people who are depressed lose interest in sex. This may be a function of the biochemistry of depression as well as of psychological factors, if that distinction holds true.

Sexual problems at a time of depression may not be the most important issue to deal with for the patient, but now that we are increasingly recommending the long-term treatment of patients who are well to prevent a recurrence of depression, the issue of impaired sexual performance becomes more important. Someone who is well needs to be able to function at all levels.

7.5 What sort of drugs cause sexual problems?

 Many drugs can cause sexual problems, including thiazides, beta-blockers, carbamazepines, cimetidine, diamorphine, digoxin, disulfiram, clofibrate, some antipsychotics as well as antidepressants. Antipsychotics specifically cause sexual impairment, partly by raising prolactin levels and also by their alpha-blocking actions and by blocking dopamine. Antidepressants appear to cause sexual impairment specifically by stimulating 5HT$_2$ neuronal pathways. Associated physical illnesses such as diabetes, multiple sclerosis and alcoholic neuropathy can of course also cause sexual problems.

7.6 Which antidepressants commonly affect libido?

 Antidepressants generally do not affect libido, and impaired libido is probably a function of low mood and drive.

The common antidepressant effects are problems in arousal, erectile problems and anorgasmia. This would appear to be primarily neuropharmacological. Most antidepressants impair sexual performance. Mirtazapine appears to be less likely to cause that difficulty, because of its unique pharmacological profile which enhances 5HT$_2$. Nefazodone was also an antidepressant which did not cause sexual impairment, but it has now been withdrawn.

7.7 Which antidepressants commonly affect orgasm and ejaculation?

 This is a common antidepressant effect, and most may impair this function. Mirtazapine appears to be uniquely less likely to impair orgasm and ejaculation because its specific pharmacological action does not impair 5HT$_2$.

This can be turned to advantage, and SSRIs are effective in treating premature ejaculation in men. They simply take a dose or two and premature ejaculation can be prevented. This is a direct pharmacological effect of the antidepressant and does not require time for the action to develop.

7.8 Which antidepressant has the best side-effect profile vis-à-vis sexual problems?

 Mirtazapine has a unique pharmacological profile, enhancing 5HT$_2$. It has been shown to cause little impairment of sexual performance. Moclobemide is low on sexual side-effects also.

7.9 What are the treatment options for drug-related sexual problems?

First an awareness for the patient that the difficulties are drug related rather than innate. This puts his or her mind at rest. In my experience many patients are happy to then tolerate this particular side-effect in favour of the benefits of not being depressed. The patient may prefer to stay on the current medication rather than change. Mirtazapine appears to cause less in the way of sexual problems because of its $5HT_2$-enhancing action. A review of the patient's need for an antidepressant overall should be undertaken, and the relative benefits and risks of stopping treatment should be considered. A reduced dose may be appropriate, and drug holidays may be considered – for example stopping the antidepressant for three or four days may enable a window of opportunity for satisfactory sexual relations. In extreme cases psychosexual therapy may be indicated, or drugs such as sildenafil may also be appropriate.

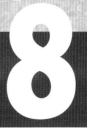

GENERAL QUESTIONS

SELECTIVE SEROTONIN REUPTAKE INHIBITORS (SSRIs)

PQ PATIENT QUESTIONS

GENERAL QUESTIONS

8.1 **GPs are being asked to diagnose and treat depression effectively, yet there are so many different drugs available it is difficult to know which one to choose. What general advice would you give about drug treatment?**

> Get to know a limited number of antidepressants well and how to use them effectively. A good guide would be to use those widely used by your local psychiatric service. This should coincide with the antidepressants that are available on your local formularies. It would be useful to have one that is slightly sedative, another that is relatively neutral, a third where the dose can be titrated up from a low starting dose to a full therapeutic dose. Possibly one with a different biochemical (e.g. SSRI/SNRI) profile could be a second-line treatment if the first-line treatment does not work. Two or three antidepressants used on a regular basis are probably sufficient. The differences in efficacy among the many antidepressants on the market are generally slight, and centre mainly on side-effect profiles rather than efficacy, but in clinical practice there are many patients who appear to benefit from one and not another antidepressant, so there appear to be differences that are hard to define from known pharmacological characteristics.
>
> Characteristics of a variety of antidepressants are given in *Table 8.1.*

8.2 **The newer antidepressants are considerably more expensive than the older tricyclics. Do you think this expense is justified in terms of safety, efficacy and compliance?**

Yes. The newer antidepressants are certainly safer both in routine practice and in overdose. They lack the cholinergic side-effects which lead to constipation and urinary problems. They lack cardiotoxicity and, with a few notable exceptions, have minimal psychomotor impairment and do not interact with alcohol. They are much less toxic than tricyclics in overdose.

The question of efficacy is less clear on direct comparison, but when the issue of compliance is added, there are distinct advantages. If patients take the full dose of medication for an adequate period of time, they are more likely to benefit from the treatment. Most newer antidepressants can be given at a therapeutically effective dose from the first day of treatment. Often one dose per day is sufficient, thus avoiding the need to titrate the dose up or for multiple dosings, both of which are a deterrent to good compliance. On that basis, efficacy is likely to be improved because of better

TABLE 8.1 Characteristics of some antidepressants

Name	Dose range daily	Type	Depression	Depression with anxiety	OCD	Panic	Social phobia	Relapse prevention	Comments
Citalopram (Cipramil)	20–60 mg	SSRI	•						
Clomipramine (Anafranil)	50–250 mg	TCA	•		•	•	•		Not in epilepsy, recent heart attack
Dothiepin/Dosulepin (Prothiaden)	75–225 mg	TCA	•	•					Pain
Escitalopram (Cipralex)	10–20 mg	SSRI	•						Tried and tested
Fluoxetine (Prozac)	20–60 mg	SSRI	•	•	•	•			Bulimia Severe PMT Double depression Premature ejaculation
L-tryptophan (Optimax)	3–6 g	Amino acid	•						EMS risk* Adjunct to treatment of severe depression
Maprotiline (Ludiomil)	25–150 mg	NaRI	•						Not sedative Probably OK for breast feeding No obvious cognitive impairment
Mirtazapine (Zispin)	15–45 mg	NaSSA	•						Sedative, hypnotic Weight gain, less sexual dysfunction

TABLE 8.1 (cont'd) Characteristics of some antidepressants

Name	Dose range daily	Type	Depression	Depression with anxiety	OCD	Panic	Social phobia	Relapse prevention	Comments
Moclobemide (Manerix)	300–600 mg	RIMA	•				•		No sexual impairment
Paroxetine (Seroxat)	20–60 mg	SSRI	•	•	•	•	•	•	PTSD
Phenelzine (Nardil)	15–45 mg	MAOI	•						Classic MAOI food and drink restrictions
Reboxetine (Edronax)	8–12 mg	NaRI	•					•	Good in fatigue
Sertraline (Lustral)	50–200 mg	SSRI	•	•	•			•	PTSD in women
Tranylcypromine (Parnate)	10–30 mg	MAOI	•						Classic MAOI food and drink restrictions
Trazodone (Molipaxin)	100–600 mg		•	•					Low CVS risk Few anticholinergic effects Sedative
Venlafaxine (Effexor)	75–375 mg	SNRI	•	•				•	Possibly more effective than other antidepressants

CVS, cardiovascular system; EMS, eosinophilia myalgia syndrome; NaRI, noradrenaline reuptake inhibitor; MAOI, monoamine oxidase inhibitor; NaSSA, noradrenergic and specific serotonergic antidepressant; OCD, obsessive compulsive disorder; PMT, premenstrual tension; PTSD, post-traumatic stress disorder; RIMA, reversible inhibitor of monoamine oxidase-A; SNRI, selective serotonin–noradrenergic reuptake inhibitor; SSRI, selective serotonin reuptake inhibitor; TCA, tricyclic antidepressant. *Hospital specialist use only.

compliance and the ability to reach the therapeutic dose early. I know there is a disagreement between GPs and psychiatrists over what constitutes an effective dose of a tricyclic.

The cost–benefit analysis of these relative advantages is more difficult to calculate, depending on who is doing the arithmetic and how much different components of the equation are valued. Some would say that money is saved by:

- better compliance, leading to greater efficacy
- less need for treatment in intensive care units following overdoses
- greater savings in getting patients back to work sooner

but a lot depends on which budget the money comes out of and how you do your arithmetic. Drug budgets are highly visible on a balance sheet, but we are doctors not accountants.

8.3 If an antidepressant does not appear to be working after a couple of months' treatment, what should I do?

The first question is whether the patient has the sort of depression that is likely to benefit from antidepressants. Sadly, antidepressants do not cure sadness, social adversity or personality disorders. You should consider whether the patient has the sort of depression that ought to benefit, namely of sufficient severity with the presence of 'biological symptoms', or is it more an 'existential depression' for which there may be no medical cure? Another common reason for therapeutic failure is a lack of compliance. Patients are often reluctant to take medication, and when they do they take it irregularly. Some GPs are often reluctant to prescribe the maximum dose of medication, whereas psychiatrists are keen to do so. It is always worth increasing the dose to the next dosage increment or even more before giving up the particular drug as ineffective. I would advocate a dosage increase before changing to another drug providing there are no side-effects. The question then is should one change to a drug of another class for example SSRI to a tricyclic or SNRI, or will another SSRI do equally well? The evidence at present is that it does not matter what antidepressant to change to, a change in medication generally confers some therapeutic benefit (10–20% chance of success) if one antidepressant does not work. Further strategies for treatment resistance (*see Box 8.1*), such as augmentation therapies with lithium, combined antidepressants, the addition of tryptophan, thyroxine or ECT, are best left in the hands of specialists, unless you feel confident in doing so yourself. (*See also Chapter 11.*)

8.4 How long should treatment last, and how should it be stopped?

Patients are unlikely to get the full benefit of an antidepressant in less than 3–4 weeks, and it sometimes takes up to 6 weeks to get the maximum

---

BOX 8.1 Treatment for resistant depression

- Addition of lithium
- ECT
- High doses of non-tricyclic antidepressant
- Addition of tri-iodothyronine (T3)
- Addition of amitriptyline
- Addition of pindolol
- Addition of dexamethasone
- Addition of lamotrigine
- High-dose tricyclics
- MAOIs and tricyclics
- Addition of buspirone
- Addition of clonazepam
- Mirtazapine
- Addition of olanzapine
- Addition of folic acid

---

benefit. If the patient has benefited from treatment, the evidence is that there is a 50% risk of relapsing in the following weeks if the antidepressant is stopped. If they continue on the medication the risk of relapse drops to about 20%. The risk of relapse generally drops to about 20% on stopping medication after 6 months – much the same as if the patient stayed on the medication. On that basis the general advice is to continue the medication for about 6 months if it has been of benefit and the side-effects are tolerable, before gradually cutting down the medication. As with everything there is a value judgement necessary, depending upon the benefit that the patient gets from the medication, whether or not they are happy to continue with it, whether they get side-effects, and the consequences of relapsing. If the patient is severely ill and has derived considerable benefit from the medication then he or she would be advised to continue the medication for longer, whereas if the therapeutic response has been marginal and the side-effects troublesome then continuing with medication may be less justified. As a rule of thumb, continue the medication for 6 months after the depression has receded.

8.5   Will some patients need to stay on medication for a longer period?

Patients with unstable conditions, where the impact of relapse is substantial, would be advised to stay on medication longer and possibly indefinitely. The evidence is that the longer patients stay on medication the less chance of relapsing. Prophylactic antidepressants appear to be of benefit in preventing recurrences, and if patients are prone to frequent relapses then they may well be happy to stay on medication indefinitely to reduce the chances of relapse. This has to be balanced against the cost in financial and personal terms of taking long-term treatment.

8.6 What are the desirable properties of an antidepressant drug?

The main requirement is that it is effective, not only in treating the acute episode but also in preventing relapse. Sadly, modern antidepressants are only about 70% effective, and we need something that is more effective than the standard preparations. Also there is a delay in establishing a full effect; a treatment that became effective in the first few days would be highly desirable. The treatment has to be safe. Fortunately modern antidepressants have side-effect profiles very similar to placebo, although every now and then something untoward occurs. Importantly, they are generally safe in overdose. The treatment should be simple to administer, ideally with a once-daily dosage. There should be no potential for abuse and no withdrawal problems. They should be free of drug interactions and should be safe not only in uncomplicated cases but also in those where there is concomitant physical illness, especially in the elderly who have cardiovascular disease and other physical ailments. Ideally of course the antidepressants should be curative, as opposed to simply suppressing symptoms, but that may be a search for the Holy Grail.

8.7 How does alcohol interact with antidepressants, and should all patients be advised not to drink at all while on treatment?

The warning about drinking alcohol while taking antidepressants is a generic one related to all categories of antidepressants. The real danger is with sedative antidepressants, where the antihistamine component of the antidepressant has an additive effect on the sedative effects of the alcohol; this can result in sedation and possible disinhibition over and above what would be expected with either compound on its own. This is a particular problem with the tricyclics and, for example, mirtazapine. The SSRIs and other more-modern compounds tend not to interact with alcohol to any significant degree, so therefore there is theoretically no harm in a patient drinking modest amounts of alcohol. Excessive amounts of alcohol or high doses of antidepressants may well be ill advised in combination, especially in emotionally unstable individuals. Patients should be advised to be careful, but there is probably no harm in a small amount of alcohol in combination with an antidepressant. The important thing is they should try it out under conditions of relative safety such as in their own home with a partner present, rather than going to a social gathering and drinking to excess and risking loss of control and social embarrassment. The answer to

the issue of whether patients who are well but remain on long-term antidepressants can indulge in social drinking is probably yes.

The very specific contraindication of Chianti for patients on MAOI therapy is dealt with in *Qs 6.5 and 6.6.*

Drug abuse is best avoided, although its effects in combination with antidepressants are generally unknown. Some SSRIs appear to reduce craving for cocaine, but this is generally an area for specialist involvement. Many depressed patients self-medicate with drugs, and many drug-abusing patients become depressed. Dual diagnosis, as it is known, where patients have a drug and psychiatric problem at the same time, is an expanding area. I am increasingly asked to see patients who have blamed aggressive or violent behaviour on their antidepressants, but in whom the likely cause is actually the effects of substantial amounts of alcohol taken at the same time by an individual with an unstable personality.

8.8   Is it better to give sedatives or antidepressants for anxiety?

Sedatives are probably contraindicated, but anxiolytics are effective in the treatment of anxiety, especially in the short term, possibly while the antidepressants begin to work. Anxiolytics such as benzodiazepines are highly effective in dealing with acute short-term crises, allowing patients the opportunity to deal with the psychological trauma and recover their composure over a few days. So, if the anxiety symptoms are likely to last for only a week or so, then probably a brief course of anxiolytics is all that is indicated. A brief course of a sedative or hypnotic may deal with a brief crisis-induced sleep problem.

If the problem is likely to be more related to a depressive illness of longer duration then the case for giving an antidepressant is stronger, but of course they take time to work and are not necessarily more effective than anxiolytics. The case for giving an antidepressant is that they do not cause dependency and are better at treating the depressive symptoms. Patients are then better able to discontinue their antidepressant medication because of the lack of withdrawal problems, whereas if they took anxiolytics they may have some withdrawal symptoms and may continue taking them in the longer term. Nevertheless benzodiazepine anxiolytics are pleasant to take and patients generally prefer taking them to taking antidepressants. There is currently still a large amount of excessive prejudice against benzodiazepines, and therefore few people would recommend prescribing them long-term to patients who are not already dependent on them. Anxiolytics are often victims of their own success.

There may be a case for prescribing benzodiazepines to cover the first few days and weeks of treatment with an antidepressant before the antidepressant effect kicks in, whereupon the aim is to tail off the benzodiazepine. In my experience patients prefer taking the benzodiazepine, and even when the antidepressants have worked they continue benzodiazepines; that has to be guarded against.

8.9 Does nicotine interact with antidepressants or have an antidepressant effect of its own?

CASE STUDY 8.1
A 26-year-old female patient with recurrent depression who was doing well on nefazodone became increasingly depressed when she gave up smoking. She improved when her treatment was changed to paroxetine.

The antidepressant effects of nicotine are probably a learned and short-term effect. Patients develop tolerance and then become dysphoric without nicotine. Some antidepressants can counteract nicotine withdrawal effects. Bupropion, an antidepressant that facilitates dopaminergic transmission, acts in this way. Others such as the SSRIs appear to be less effective in this respect. Clinical experience shows that, in patients who become depressed when they give up cigarette smoking and who can benefit from an antidepressant for their depressive symptoms, bupropion would be the obvious choice, although the treatment of depression is not a licensed indication. I have seen patients who have been helped in dealing with nicotine withdrawal by taking an antidepressant, and it is certainly worth a try.

8.10 Do patients become dependent on antidepressants in the same way that they may become dependent on benzodiazepines?

No. Antidepressants have a different mechanism of action from benzodiazepines and do not act on the alcohol–GABA–benzodiazepine receptor complex. They are not associated with the classic tolerance and withdrawal syndrome associated with sedative hypnotic compounds. Patients can become clinically reliant on antidepressants to prevent recurrences and relapses. There may be some level of psychological habituation. The suggestion that long-term antidepressant consumption can make patients more liable to relapse on stopping antidepressants is an interesting notion and one without real evidence to support it. The Committee on Safety of Medicines tells us there is little evidence, from spontaneous reporting, of dependency. Other published literature and usage data suggest that SSRIs and related drugs are not drugs of dependence.

Withdrawal reactions have been reported with SSRIs. These commonly include symptoms of dizziness, paraesthesia, headaches, anxiety and nausea. These symptoms are distinct from a recurrence of depression. They tend to last a few days only. Because of this, abrupt discontinuation of treatment with antidepressants should be avoided. It is best to cut down the medication over a matter of days to minimize any withdrawal symptoms.

8.11 Is there any point in switching a patient from one SSRI to another SSRI and, if so, what precautions should I take?

Ideally you should withdraw the first SSRI and then start the replacement. The reduction should be over 2–4 weeks. An alternative strategy would be to halve the dose of one SSRI and substitute it for the half dose of the other one, thereby cross tapering. There should not be any problem. There are two reasons for switching from one SSRI to another. The first would be because of side-effects. Providing the side-effects are not general to SSRIs as a class (headaches and nausea) but specific to a particular drug, then that might be a reason for changing. The alternative reason would be lack of efficacy, and it is as valid to change to another SSRI as it is to change to an entirely different type of antidepressant.

8.12 If I decide to switch a patient from an SSRI to an NaSSA or vice versa, what precautions should I take?

This is best done by cautious cross tapering, increasing the dose of one while cautiously reducing the other. The same applies whichever way you go. There is logic in switching to a different class of antidepressant if the switch is instigated because of an inadequate therapeutic response or side-effects. Noradrenergic and specific serotonergic antidepressants (NaSSAs) theoretically have an additional mode of action, by inhibiting the uptake of noradrenaline (norepinephrine), compared with an SSRI and therefore might work when the latter has not, but definitive evidence for this is lacking.

Similar considerations apply when switching between an SSRI and an SNRI.

8.13 If I decide to switch a patient from an MAOI to an SSRI or vice versa, what precautions should I take?

Combining SSRIs and traditional MAOIs is extremely dangerous and can result in fatal reactions. Great caution needs to be exercised if a switch is contemplated. Two weeks have to be left after stopping MAOIs before introducing any other antidepressant. Two weeks have to be left after stopping an SSRI (5 weeks for fluoxetine) before starting an MAOI. This is a procedure best left in the hands of a specialist. It usually entails gradually tapering down one antidepressant in someone who is not responding, and giving a 2-week drug holiday before starting on another antidepressant, which may take several weeks to work. This means that the patient will be without effective treatment for several weeks and will need support during this time.

8.14 If I decide to switch a patient from an MAOI to a tricyclic or vice versa, what precautions should I take?

This can also be hazardous, and great caution needs to be exercised. Adding a tricyclic antidepressant in a patient already on an MAOI can result in a fatal interaction, with the dramatic 'serotonin syndrome' of hyperpyrexia, fits, elevated blood pressure and death. *Adding a tricyclic thus to an MAOI is absolutely contraindicated.* Adding an MAOI to a tricyclic is acceptable under some circumstances. If the tricyclic is one of the secondary amines such as dosulepin (dothiepin), amitriptyline or trimipramine, then it may be clinically appropriate to add phenelzine carefully, one of the older treatments for resistant depression. If, however, the patient is taking imipramine the procedure may be hazardous. Phenelzine is the MAOI to use. It is best to avoid tranylcypromine. Again this is a procedure best left in the hands of the dwindling number of psychiatrists experienced in these matters.

8.15 If I decide to switch a patient from a tricyclic to an SSRI or vice versa, what precautions should I take?

 This should not pose a problem. Ideally, cross-tapering cautiously with a low dose of tricyclic added to the SSRI or vice versa and then gradually increasing the dose would be the best way forward.

Appendix 5 gives, for a variety of antidepressants, details of precautions to take when switching or stopping the drugs.

8.16 What is the serotonin syndrome, and how may it be avoided?

 This condition is characterized by restlessness, sweating, tremor, shivering, muscle spasms, confusion, convulsions and ultimately death (*Box 8.2*). It classically occurs with the combination of MAOIs and SSRIs. It can occur to a lesser degree if for example the dose of an SSRI is too high or if it is combined with lithium or L-tryptophan, both drugs that increase the functional amounts of serotonin in the system. In its milder form it is treated by drug discontinuation; in its more severe forms it is a medical emergency and needs symptomatic treatment often in an intensive-care unit.

8.17 What are cholinergic rebound effects?

 These are symptoms of mild anxiety, restlessness, possible insomnia with nightmares, tiredness, dizziness and headaches. There might be nausea and vomiting. These symptoms are generally short lived and, when caused by the withdrawal of antidepressants, are at the mild end of the spectrum.

BOX 8.2 The serotonin syndrome

Neurological symptoms: myoclonus, nystagmus, headache, tremor, rigidity, seizures
Mental state changes: irritability, confusion, agitation, coma
Other symptoms: hyperpyrexia, cardiac arrhythmias, death

8.18 Do some drugs cause symptoms even after they have been discontinued?

Once a drug has left the body, and the body has readjusted by homeostasis, then all effects caused by the antidepressant should be over. The obvious exception is when some permanent damage is done by a side-effect, such as agranulocytosis or hepatic necrosis or some other dramatic drug-specific effect. Some patients complain of long-term withdrawal effects lasting several months and years, especially following the use of benzodiazepine tranquillizers. In my experience this is more a function of a return of the underlying illness rather than a prolonged withdrawal reaction or specific side-effect caused by a drug.

8.19 Can bupropion, the anti-smoking drug, be prescribed to a patient who is already taking antidepressants?

This should only be done cautiously, because of the risk of causing epileptiform convulsions. Antidepressants lower the threshold for seizures, and two will do so more than one. It is a rare problem. On the other hand adding bupropion to another antidepressant is a known treatment for resistant depression and may actually enhance the therapeutic effect.

8.20 How can I help patients deal with the stigma of taking antidepressants?

Sadly there is a stigma both about being depressed and having mental illness in general and secondly about the consequential need for antidepressant medication. The first stigma to deal with is that of mental illness. The Royal College of Psychiatrists is currently running a 5-year campaign entitled 'Changing Minds: Every Family in the Land' dealing with precisely this issue. Information is available from them and of course their website (www.rcpsych.ac.uk). It is helpful for patients to know that they are not alone in their affliction. An explanation that maybe one in ten people will suffer depression at some time in their lives goes some way to make patients realize they are not unique. Getting in touch with self-help groups and providing patients with helpful user-friendly information sheets is a useful route. The most helpful factor is allowing the patients to realize that someone close to them, possibly at work, has also suffered from depression and recovered. Helping patients realize that their depression is not a sign of weakness, failure or inadequacy is important, although these are precisely the emotions that their depression will conjure up.

Some patients feel that it is the taking of the antidepressant itself that is in some way stigmatizing. Having to stand in a pharmacy and admit to yourself and to others that you are depressed and in some way inadequate is something people do not like doing. Patients then translate their anxiety about taking antidepressants into fears of addiction, dependency and the belief that they have no willpower and need to resort to external means to overcome their problem. Ultimately, reassurance, patience and encouragement constitute the essential support needed in helping people deal with their anxieties.

TRICYCLIC ANTIDEPRESSANTS (TCAS)

8.21 How do TCAs work, and are they effective?

The leading theory to explain the biological basis of depression has been the monoamine hypothesis. According to this, depression is due to or mediated by a deficiency in one or another of three biogenic monoamine neurotransmitters: serotonin, noradrenaline (norepinephrine) or dopamine. Tricyclic antidepressants act by increasing the functional amount of these monoamines in the synaptic cleft by blocking their reuptake once they have

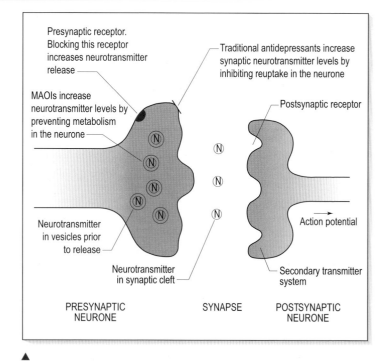

Fig. 8.1 Sites of antidepressant action.

been released (*see Fig. 8.1*). There may then be a postsynaptic down-regulation, which is probably the next step in antidepressant action.

Tricyclics are the traditional antidepressants and are as effective as any other, giving an overall efficacy of about 70% as opposed to about 30% for placebo (by whatever means this is measured).

8.22 Are they more or less effective than other antidepressants, particularly the SSRIs?

In general in head-to-head clinical trials they are as effective as SSRIs. There are some suggestions that clomipramine may perhaps be slightly more powerful, but this is not a consistent finding. How this then translates into everyday clinical practice is a more complicated question. Because some of the older antidepressants have side-effects and need dosage titration and multiple dosings, they are more complicated to give and there is greater room for patients to have subtherapeutic doses or to manifest poor compliance. On that basis they may ultimately be less effective than the more palatable, easier to administer, newer antidepressants.

8.23 Why are TCAs so dangerous in overdose?

Tricyclics are for the most part 'dirty drugs', having actions on many different neuronal systems and pathways beyond the primary amine-reuptake-blocking action. In overdose, these secondary pharmacological actions become important, the most important being the quinidine-like action upon the heart that can result in ventricular arrhythmias and other cardiac complications. The anticholinergic action can be excitatory to the heart, there is some alpha-blockade resulting in hypotension, and the antihistamine action can potentiate other sedatives, especially alcohol, resulting in deeper comas and complications associated with that. Some antidepressants are epileptogenic, and this can result in fits especially in susceptible individuals.

8.24 Are TCAs effective in treating both depression and anxiety?

Yes. To what degree this is a function of the sedative actions or their specific neurotransmitter profile is uncertain. The antidepressants which markedly block serotonin reuptake, such as clomipramine, have demonstrated efficacy in the treatment of obsessive compulsive disorder. They also appear to be effective in phobic states and bulimia. Imipramine has been demonstrated to be effective in panic disorders, although the dosage necessary can be quite low. Tricyclic antidepressants and the newer classes of antidepressants are effective in treating a broad spectrum of mood disorders and allied conditions.

8.25 What are the major side-effects encountered by the patient taking TCAs?

 The common anticholinergic side-effects are a dry mouth, constipation, urinary retention and impotence. Sweating, blurred vision, confusion, problems with narrow-angle glaucoma, and cardiovascular side-effects – tachycardia, arrhythmias, postural hypotension and syncope, cardiomyopathy, cardiac failure and ECG changes – are rare but serious. Other side-effects include seizures, tremor, weight gain and, rarely, agranulocytosis.

The side-effects are primarily the result of unwanted actions on physiological systems unrelated to the treatment of depression, namely anticholinergic actions, alpha-blocking actions, quinidine-like actions and antihistamine effects (*Box 8.3*). In addition there are the idiosyncratic effects.

8.26 What are the toxic effects encountered in overdose?

 Toxic effects are cardiac arrhythmias, cardiac arrest, ECG changes (*Fig. 8.2*), prolongation of QT interval, postural hypotension, epileptic seizures, hyperreflexia, mydriasis, coma and death.

The major effects in overdose are caused by the atropine-like effects, neurological effects and cardiovascular effects. In addition there is the sedation caused by the antihistamine function.

The important features and potentially fatal effects are cardiac arrhythmias and conduction defects – an important diagnostic feature distinguishing tricyclic overdoses from others. This can lead to ventricular fibrillation and cardiac arrest. There can be hypertension followed by hypotension. Epileptic seizures and hyperpyrexia can occur. Sedation and seizures can result in inhalation pneumonitis, another potential cause of death. There is often a delay of some days before the fatal arrhythmias

---

BOX 8.3 Unwanted effects of TCAs at secondary sites of pharmacological action

Antihistamine H1 – weight gain, drowsiness
Anticholinergic – constipation, blurred vision, dry mouth, drowsiness, urinary retention, glaucoma, confusion – especially in the elderly, potency problems
Quinidine – cardiac arrhythmias
Alpha-1 – hypotension, dizziness, drowsiness
Non-specific – epileptiform convulsions, agranulocytosis (rare)

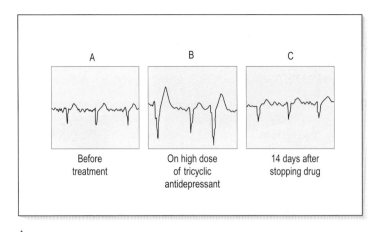

▲

Fig. 8.2 ECG changes in a patient on a tricyclic antidepressant.

become manifest, so it may be dangerous to discharge the patient too soon following an overdose.

8.27 How many deaths are caused by TCA overdoses per year in the UK?

Before the widespread introduction of the more modern and safer antidepressants, approximately one person per day on average died of antidepressant overdose (350 per year). This has to be seen in the context of about 1330 deaths annually as a result of self-poisoning and approximately 6000 suicides annually. Nevertheless the National Suicide Prevention Strategy for England recommends the promotion of safer prescribing of antidepressants to help combat the current epidemic of suicide. About 5% of suicides were caused by tricyclic antidepressants, a notable figure in an identifiable high-risk group (*see Fig. 8.3*). Tricyclic overdoses are of course often taken in combination with other drugs which complicate the picture considerably.

8.28 Why are TCAs used to treat neuralgia and chronic pain in the absence of depression?

Tricyclic antidepressants have an enhancing effect on the descending bulbo-spinal 5HT-mediated analgesic pathway to the dorsal horn. Thus theoretically they have an analgesic action independent of any antidepressant effect. An analgesic effect of amitriptyline has been shown

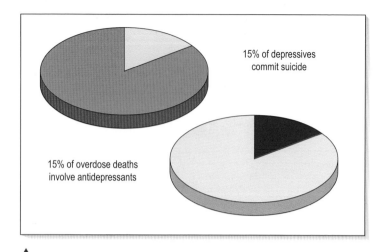

15% of depressives
commit suicide

15% of overdose deaths
involve antidepressants

Fig. 8.3 Depression and suicide. (Data from West R 1991 Depression. Office of Health Economics, London.)

convincingly in some neuropathic pains, notably post-herpetic neuralgia. The SSRIs are less effective. The doses of amitriptyline used are usually far below what would be an effective antidepressant dose. There may be some benefit from the mild sedation or anxiolytic action also. There may also be a strong placebo effect. Antidepressants also have an effect on migraine headaches by blocking the uptake of 5HT into the cerebral blood vessels, which is so important in the causation of migraine, as well as the specific action on the $5HT_{1D}$ receptor.

8.29 I believe that dosulepin is the most widely prescribed TCA. Why is this?

SSRIs are certainly the most widely prescribed antidepressants when initiating new treatment, but tricyclics remain widely prescribed in patients who are established on long-term treatment and who are happy with it. Indeed patients should not be switched from one medication to another if there is no problem. 'If it ain't bust, don't fix it'. Tricyclics are also widely used by pain specialists.

8.30 Is trazodone different from other TCAs, and when is it most useful?

Trazodone is not a tricyclic. It has a 'unique structure' and mode of action, being mainly a $5HT_2$ antagonist as well as performing as an uptake inhibitor.

It is low in cardiotoxicity and anticholinergic side-effects, but produces a higher incidence of drowsiness because of its antihistamine properties and causes nausea. On that basis it is useful for agitated depression and also in patients with insomnia because of its sedative qualities.

8.31 Are the second-generation TCAs, e.g. lofepramine and dosulepin, any different from amitriptyline?

Lofepramine is a tricyclic similar to imipramine but with a more favourable side-effect profile. It appears to be uniquely safe in overdose and has less in the way of cholinergic cardiovascular side-effects. It is mainly a noradrenergic reuptake inhibitor and therefore is categorized as an SNRI (selective serotonin–noradrenergic reuptake inhibitor). Dosulepin (dothiepin) is an analogue of amitriptyline. It is generally lower on side-effects but reputed to be more lethal in overdose.

8.32 Is lofepramine recommended for any particular type of depression?

Yes, it is particularly useful in the elderly where cardiac side-effects and hypotension may be an issue, and also in potentially suicidal patients. It is less good for agitated patients. It has a slightly stimulating action. The advantages are that it can be titrated upwards from 70 mg to the full dose of 210 mg or even more if necessary.

8.33 For whom is mianserin suitable, and are any special precautions necessary?

Mianserin was generally safe in overdose and somewhat sedative, but the need for a full blood count every month made it too cumbersome to give, and it has been withdrawn. Mirtazapine is effectively a newer, safer version which has superseded mianserin.

MONOAMINE OXIDASE INHIBITORS (MAOIs)

8.34 How do MAOIs work?

The classical MAOIs phenelzine, tranylcypromine and iproniazid work by inhibiting the enzyme inside neurones that breaks down amine neurotransmitters after they have been reabsorbed from the synapse (*see Fig. 8.1*). By doing this they increase the amount of other antidepressants available for release. This action is generally different from that of tricyclics, which block the reuptake of neurotransmitters from the synapse or block the presynaptic receptors which stimulate the release of neurotransmitters. MAOIs tend to work on all of the amine neurotransmitters: serotonin, noradrenaline and dopamine. The newer, reversible inhibitors of monoamine oxidase-A (RIMAs), supposedly act in a similar way, but do not have the same risk of drug interaction and the cheese effect, since they do not inhibit the MAO in the bowel and are reversible.

8.35 Are they effective antidepressants, and when should they be used?

In general MAOIs are seen as less effective than the standard tricyclic-type reuptake inhibitors. The view is that they are more suitable for 'atypical depression' where anxiety and phobic anxiety, obsessional and hysterical symptoms are more prominent. They can be used in resistant depression when other antidepressants have been tried and failed. They are often useful in chronic anxiety disorders where depression is a lesser feature. There was a vogue for combining phenelzine with amitriptyline, trimipramine or dosulepin (dothiepin) as a treatment for resistant depression. In general, however, partly because they are no longer being marketed and partly because of the almost unacceptable side-effect profile, mostly to do with the highly dangerous 'cheese reaction' or hypertensive crisis in combination with other drugs, they have virtually stopped being used outside of the hands of specialists experienced in their use.

The newer generation of RIMAs would appear to be very much safer, but sadly in my experience moclobemide, the only commercially available RIMA, is not very effective, despite the published evidence to the contrary.

8.36 What are the main drug and food interactions with this group?

The main drug interaction is with tyramine, which is present in protein and is released when the protein decomposes. This is found in cheese (decomposed milk), hung game (decomposed meat), Marmite (decomposed yeast), and a whole host of other exotic foods (*see Box 8.4*). Although the list is exhaustive and frightening, most patients find it relatively easy to deal with the dietary restrictions, which are really quite straightforward. Sympathomimetic amines are also to be discouraged, as should other amines such as phenylethylamine (present in chocolate). MAOIs interfere with the metabolism of pethidine, and on that basis this drug should not be given. There is a dramatic and highly dangerous interaction with antidepressants, especially SSRIs, which are quite likely to result in the fatal hypertensive and hyperpyrexial 'serotonin syndrome' (*see Q. 8.16*).

8.37 What advice should be given to patients starting MAOI treatment?

Patients should be warned of the dietary restrictions in detail and given a dietary warning card, which if not available immediately can be added to the prescription and supplied by the pharmacist. The risks to patients are very small providing they obey the dietary restrictions, which really come

---

BOX 8.4 Monoamine oxidase inhibitors – important potential dietary and drug interactions

Dietary[a]

Cheese
Bovril/Oxo/Marmite
Pickled herring
Broad bean pods
Food going 'off', e.g. offal/game/fish
Alcohol, especially Chianti or fortified wines

Drugs

Sympathomimetics (as in nasal decongestants)
Tricyclics (e.g. clomipramine) and SSRIs
Amphetamines
Fenfluramine
L-dopa/dopamine
Pethidine
Barbiturates

---

[a]An early warning symptom is a throbbing headache indicating a potential, severe rise in blood pressure. The wide range of possible interactions means that practitioners should always check in the *British National Formulary* and warn patients as to what they eat and the risks of other medications (e.g. anaesthetics).

---

down to avoiding cheese and Marmite. They are also a function of how much tyramine-containing food they eat, and not all patients get bad reactions. An occasional glass of white wine or two does not appear to be harmful, only heavy red wines (which are made from the whole grape, including the skin). Drug combinations should be avoided. If patients experience really bad headaches then they should go to the local casualty department or GP surgery immediately and have their blood pressure checked as a matter of urgency. Chlorpromazine 50 mg is a good alpha-blocker for immediate help in lowering the blood pressure, before giving more-intensive hypotensive treatments if needed.

8.38 I find the drug and food interactions with MAOIs rather daunting; hence should I prescribe them? Am I denying my patients a useful treatment or should this group of drugs only be initiated by psychiatrists?

They should only be initiated by doctors experienced in giving them. In experienced hands they are not a big problem. In my view they are often very effective in the properly selected patients where other treatments seem not to work as well; some patients are probably being denied useful treatment when other treatments have failed. Because of their side-effect profile I would only see them as 'third-line treatments' after other avenues have been exhausted. If they do prove effective, patients often need to stay on them indefinitely, and sometimes tolerance occurs and the dose needs to be increased in time. Occasional drug holidays are needed to let the tolerance wear off and the patient to start at a more modest dose again.

8.39 What are the problems encountered when changing a patient's medication from an MAOI to another antidepressant or vice versa?

> Important considerations in this regard are discussed in *Qs 8.13 and 8.14*.

8.40 I have come across patients who have been prescribed MAOIs as well as TCAs – surely this is rather dangerous?

This treatment – starting a patient on a TCA and an MAOI together and slowly increasing the dose – in experienced hands is regarded by some as more effective than either treatment on its own. If anything, combining tricyclics with MAOIs protects against the cheese reaction. Provided that a sedative tricyclic and not an SSRI or imipramine is used, and ideally phenelzine is the MAOI, then the risks are relatively low. NB: Adding a TCA in a patient *who is already on an MAOI* is potentially *fatal*.

8.41 What are RIMAs and how do they differ from conventional MAOIs?

There is only one commercially available RIMA: moclobemide. RIMAs differ from traditional MAOIs in being selective for MAO(A) and also being immediately reversible and competitive with tyramine; by contrast, traditional MAOIs inhibit MAO(A) and MAO(B) for a period of weeks, and, when the drug is stopped, the enzyme levels take time to be restored. MAO(A) is the enzyme involved in the breakdown of neurotransmitters in the neurones and the one important for the treatment of depression. MAO(B) is found in the liver and gut wall, where it normally is protective and prevents the influx of tyramine into the systemic circulation where it can cause hypertensive problems. RIMAs do not affect the gut and liver MAO(B), which can still act in its protective function against the tyramine, but inhibit the neuronal MAO(A).

In addition the action of MAO(A) on the enzymes that metabolize neurotransmitters is competitive. And so if a competitor is present it stops the action of moclobemide immediately. Selegiline is a selective MAO(B) inhibitor used in the treatment of parkinsonism.

8.42 When should RIMAs be used, and are they as effective as conventional MAOIs?

RIMAs are generally not to be compared directly with conventional MAOIs but to antidepressants generally (according to the manufacturers). Although the research data suggest they are as effective as standard antidepressants, the overall impression is that they are not. They appear to be very low in side-effects, and on that basis can be used in patients who are intolerant to other antidepressants. Generally the dose needs to be increased to the upper limit of the range before any real efficacy is noted. Moclobemide is indicated for the treatment of social phobia. It is also useful in the elderly who are less able to tolerate side-effects of other antidepressants. RIMAs would appear to be less powerful as anxiolytics than conventional MAOIs.

8.43 Are RIMAs any safer in overdose or in interaction with conventional MAOIs?

The answer is yes. They are relatively safe in overdose and because they are displaced by tyramine and other amines from the enzyme systems, when challenged by hazardous amines they are removed from the system and therefore tend not to interact with other drugs.

8.44 Is it easier to change a patient's treatment from or to a RIMA than from or to an MAOI?

Yes, although the same cautions should apply. It should not be necessary, as it is for a conventional MAOI, to wait for 2 weeks after stopping a RIMA to allow the enzymes to recover – a few days should be sufficient. Adding a tricyclic to a RIMA needs 24 hours free of the RIMA. Adding a RIMA to a tricyclic is probably not hazardous, but caution dictates a gap of about 48 hours before gradually introducing the RIMA.

SELECTIVE SEROTONIN REUPTAKE INHIBITORS (SSRIs)

8.45 How does this group of antidepressants work?

They work in the same way that other antidepressants work: by increasing functional amounts of serotonin (5HT), one of the principal neurotransmitters involved in mood regulation, in the brain. They differ from other antidepressants in effectively only boosting levels of serotonin and not other neurotransmitters, many of which are responsible for side-effects. They are therefore 'cleaner' and more specific than other antidepressants.

8.46 When should they be used?

They are currently the medication of first choice in the treatment of depression. They have superseded the tricyclic antidepressants because of their greater tolerability and therefore ease of administration, enabling patients to get to a therapeutic dose without the need to titrate it upwards. They are generally not sedative, which can be troublesome for some patients. They lack the quinidine-like and anticholinergic effects of tricyclics, which can cause problems in those with cardiovascular disease, glaucoma and bladder problems, especially in the elderly. They are safer in overdose. Like tricyclics, many have a broad spectrum of therapeutic activity, including diagnoses such as panic disorder, OCD, bulimia and prevention of relapse of depression. They also have efficacy in the premenstrual syndrome – where they appear to have a different mode of action, as they work within a few days of being taken. Not all SSRIs have the same spectrum of licensed indications.

The suggestion that some TCAs, such as clomipramine, may be more effective than SSRIs is a possibility but relatively unimportant in normal clinical practice.

8.47 Are they (a) more effective and (b) safer in overdose than the older TCAs?

Although SSRIs are no more effective than TCAs in clinical trials, in clinical practice it is easier to get patients onto full therapeutic doses of an SSRI because there is no need to titrate the dose up, or if titration is desirable then there are fewer steps necessary to achieve a full therapeutic dose. Also patients are more likely to comply with the full dose because of a relative lack of side-effects, and on that basis they should prove more effective because patients are more likely to take them appropriately. SSRIs are of course much safer than tricyclics in overdose because they lack the sedative and quinidine-like adrenergic stimulating effects which can be cardiotoxic.

8.48 What are the main side-effects of this group of drugs?

 Headaches, GI side-effects and sexual dysfunction are the main adverse effects. Although they lack the sedative and anticholinergic side-effects of tricyclics, the most prominent and troublesome side-effects are headache and nausea, which can occur in the first few days of treatment. They may occasionally be so severe as to result in discontinuation of treatment. Another troublesome side-effect occurring in the first 24 hours of treatment is an increase in anxiety symptoms, which again can stop treatment. This is best overcome by a gradual upward titration of the dose, warning the patient it may occur, and possibly covering the first day or so of treatment with a few benzodiazepine tablets. Sexual dysfunction is a problem in prolonged use. Whereas this may not be an issue while treating an acute depressive episode, it becomes a serious issue while keeping people well long-term on prophylactic treatment. Sexual dysfunction (anorgasmia, reduced arousal and lack of libido) is a dose-related effect and can be minimized by titrating the dose down. It appears to be a specific SSRI effect and may be less of a problem with non-SSRI antidepressants. (*See also Chapter 7.*)

8.49 What was the first SSRI to be used in the UK, and did it have any particular beneficial or adverse effects?

Zimeledine (Zelmid) was the first SSRI, introduced in 1981. It was withdrawn shortly after its introduction because of a rare but serious Guillain–Barré type syndrome. The next to be introduced was fluoxetine (Prozac) in the late 1980s. At the time it was revolutionary in its selectivity and specificity. One of its characteristics was its very long half-life. It is possible that the dose at which it was introduced was too high. On that basis it probably resulted in effective doses even if the patient missed one or two capsules every week, thus improving compliance and efficacy. The problem was that, if one wanted to switch from Prozac to another antidepressant, there had to be a long washout period. It turns out, however, that the long half-life appears to be protective against withdrawal reactions. Prozac was the legendary forerunner of the other SSRIs, primarily because it caught the public imagination in America, which had been very much behind the UK in the introduction of more-modern antidepressants. With the Americans' love of new things and with skilful marketing, it achieved a phenomenal breakthrough and cult status early on.

8.50 Introduced in the UK in 1989, fluoxetine (Prozac) is the best-known drug in this group. What are its main advantages and disadvantages?

Fluoxetine is simple to take. One capsule a day should suffice, and missing the odd dose may not affect the therapeutic outcome. It is relatively low on side-effects and is generally not sedating. It may even have a mild stimulating effect due to an amphetamine-like action. The main disadvantage is that some patients experience GI side-effects.

Prozac has become a victim of its own success, and this success has brought claims of harm made by the 'Victims of Prozac' who allege that fluoxetine can drive them into violent, suicidal and homicidal acts. I do not believe these claims to be founded in reality, but they have entered into popular mythology. The myth has now spread to paroxetine.

8.51 Some people have been on Prozac for many years – indeed someone has written a book about their experiences on the drug. Does this mean that we should be wary of prescribing it because it is hard to come off, or do some people need lifelong treatment for their depression?

Several books have been written about Prozac (*see Box 8.5*). Prozac reached cult status not only as a lifestyle-enhancing drug and happiness pill, but also as an example of how pharmaceutical companies would manipulate our minds and beliefs for profit. The general view is that depressive illnesses are relatively long-term conditions with an average duration of about 18 months per cycle (*Fig. 8.4*). Therefore treating a single episode for a few weeks and then stopping the drug is associated with a strong risk of early relapse. From a psychiatric point of view we usually encourage patients to take the antidepressant for as long as possible.

Beyond the statistical risk that long-term antidepressant consumption reduces the risk of relapse by about five-fold, there is also the less clear issue of 'kindling', where every depressive relapse makes it more likely that there will be further episodes. If this is true then there is a strong case for treating depression vigorously and long term rather than the somewhat haphazard approach we adopt today. Also there is a lot to be said for allowing patients to get used to the experience of feeling well rather than being right on the edge of a recurrence of depressive symptoms. This has a psychological benefit. Being well also allows patients to deal with the therapeutic issues surrounding their illnesses either through formal therapy or through living a healthy lifestyle. On that basis I take the view that it is good to take antidepressants for somewhat longer than is absolutely necessary rather than for too short a time.

BOX 8.5 Some books written about Prozac

- *Prozac Nation*
- *Potatoes not Prozac*
- *Listening to Prozac*
- *Plato not Prozac*
- *Better than Prozac*
- *Prozac Backlash*
- *Prozac Diary*
- *Prozac: Panacea or Pandora*
- *Prozac on the Couch*
- *Natural Prozac*
- *Beyond Prozac*

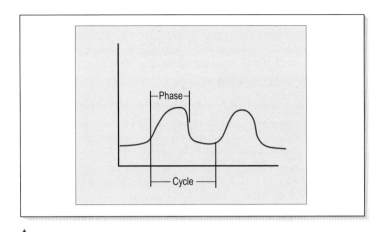

▲

Fig. 8.4 Cyclic pattern of recurrent depression.

The issue of whether SSRIs are 'addictive' has recently been raised. Addiction is a dramatic word used when people take substances against medical advice and to their ultimate detriment. This is not the case with antidepressants. Some patients may experience withdrawal symptoms, and there may be some small element of physiological dependency. This can be overcome by gradually tailing off the dose over a couple of weeks. Some patients become dependent upon the idea of feeling well. Some patients need lifelong treatment for their depression, others become reliant upon the use of a pill, which is probably not therapeutically indicated. As with all powerful treatments, the risks and benefits need to be evaluated, especially if consigning someone to a long-term treatment that has cost and health implications. There may be a case for seeking a specialist opinion if there are concerns about long-term use.

8.52 Some SSRIs are easier to stop than others. Why is this so? How should SSRIs be withdrawn at the end of the treatment period?

SSRIs with short half-lives appear to cause more withdrawal reactions than do longer-acting ones. Most notably paroxetine has been tarred with the withdrawal reaction label. Fluoxetine, with its long half-life, seems not to have this problem. The way to overcome withdrawal problems is to cut down the dose gradually, by reducing the dose to half a tablet daily and thereafter half on alternate days over a 2-week period. If withdrawal reactions are really a problem there may be a case for switching to fluoxetine first (because of its long half-life) and then gradually withdrawing, or switching to the liquid form of the SSRI and titrating the dose downwards in more gradual steps. The patient should be warned that any symptoms experienced will be transient and will be at their maximum in the day or two after stopping medication. They are not an indication that the patient is about to relapse.

8.53 What are the main advantages and disadvantages of sertraline?

Sertraline came in 50 mg tablets, and the initial recommendation was not to increase the dose beyond 150 mg. More recently dose increases have been allowed up to 200 mg. As well as being indicated for the treatment of depression, including associated anxiety, it has the additional licensed indication for the treatment of OCD in adults and children. It is also licensed for the treatment of PTSD in women but, interestingly, not men. It is generally well tolerated by patients, low on side-effects and suitable for patients who have had recent cardiac disease or strokes. There is little interaction with other drugs. The disadvantage is an uncertain dose range. There remains debate as to whether all the SSRIs are essentially the same, or whether there are distinct differences between them. There is evidence that, if one SSRI does not work, 20% of patients will respond to the prescription of a different SSRI, and so they may not all be quite the same after all. Whether this relates to differential effects on the subclass of serotonin receptors or some other reason is unknown. (*See also Table 8.1.*)

8.54 I had a patient who only felt well on 200 mg of sertraline a day, yet I believe that this dose is not licensed for long-term use. Have you any comment to make on this?

It is well known that some patients only respond to higher doses of anti-depressants. Sertraline was only licensed for short-term use at higher doses, although that licence has now been changed and 200 mg is quite acceptable even for long-term use if clinically indicated. It is very common for treatments to be used outside their licensed indications in psychiatric practice. Licensing is about commercial and regulatory issues, but many patients do not fit into neat categories in their clinical needs and therapeutic responses.

8.55 The most recent SSRI to be introduced has been citalopram. Does it have any particular advantages over other, older SSRIs?

Citalopram is clean and effective and used in cases where there is the potential for drug interactions. Citalopram is metabolized by a different set of enzymes of the cytochrome system (the enzyme system involved in drug metabolism). There is therefore less potential for drug interactions with citalopram than with other antidepressants, which may saturate the enzymes and impede their ability to deal with both drugs at the same time. The more recent version of citalopram (escitalopram) has recently been launched. This is the L-form of the racemic mixture of citalopram, which is the pharmacologically active component of the mixture. On that basis it is a purified form of citalopram. Trials data suggest it is slightly more effective than the older citalopram, but this is probably of limited clinical relevance.

8.56 What are dual-action SSRIs, and how do they work?

Dual-action SSRIs work by not only blocking the reuptake of serotonin at the synaptic cleft but also by blocking presynaptic $5HT_2$ receptors, thereby enhancing 5HT transmission. For example mirtazapine blocks $5HT_2$ and enhances 5HT transmission in that way. These drugs appear to have less in the way of the 'fierce' $5HT_2$ side-effects such as nausea and headache (*see Box 8.6*). Whether this translates into any relevant clinical advantage or not is open to speculation.

BOX 8.6 Effects of stimulation of key 5HT receptor subtypes

Presynaptic $5HT_{1A}$

Classic SSRI antidepressant effects
– anti-anxiety
– anti-panic
– anti-OCD
– anti-appetite

$5HT_2$

Classic SSRI side-effects
– agitation
– akathisia
– anxiety
– panic attacks
– insomnia
– sexual dysfunction

$5HT_{1D}$

Anti-migraine

$5HT_3$

Nausea
Diarrhoea
Headaches

(Noradrenaline)

Controls release of 5HT

8.57 Is there any advantage in prescribing nefazodone, a dual-action SSRI?

Nefazodone has recently been withdrawn in the UK, primarily because no one was prescribing it. Nefazodone had a presynaptic $5HT_2$ blocking action, enhancing 5HT transmission, as well as being a 5HT reuptake inhibitor. Its reduced side-effect profile gave it unique qualities, namely a lack of sexual impairment and an enhancement of natural sleep. Unfortunately it was a relatively weak antidepressant requiring large doses for an effective therapeutic action, and the doses had to be titrated up. It was never a commercial success, probably because it was not a very good antidepressant despite its complex pharmacology.

8.58 What are SNRIs, and what are their advantages?

SNRIs are selective serotonin–noradrenergic reuptake inhibitors. They act on a different neurotransmitter system to the SSRIs. They boost levels of noradrenaline, as opposed to serotonin, in the synaptic cleft. They may therefore be effective in specific forms of depression where SSRIs are less effective, although the case for that is not very compelling. They do have a different spectrum of side-effects. Sexual impairment is less of an issue, and they appear to be more energizing.

8.59 What are NaSSAs, and when are they useful?

They are noradrenergic and specific serotonergic antidepressants. An example is mirtazapine, with its complex actions as an α_2 antagonist with potent HT_2-, HT_3- and antihistamine-antagonist properties. The main difference between this and other antidepressants is again in the side-effect profile. Mirtazapine is notably sedative and promotes a healthy appetite and weight gain. These effects may be advantages or disadvantages. It is otherwise an effective antidepressant.

8.60 Reboxetine is a noradrenaline reuptake inhibitor. What advantage does that offer over the older SSRIs?

The main difference is that it boosts noradrenaline in preference to other neurotransmitters. This may then translate into a different spectrum of activity for different subclasses of depression. Sadly, despite 30 years of research, there is little to suggest that particular types of depression are responsive to different types of antidepressant, and, on that basis, finding the right antidepressant for the individual patient remains a matter of trial and error. There is some evidence that reboxetine is more effective than other antidepressants, but again whether this is clinically relevant or not is open to speculation. Overall it is good to have a spectrum of pharmacological activities that at least allows the clinician to try a different class of antidepressant if there is a lack of response to the drug of first choice. For example, if an SSRI does not work there is a strong case for switching to a different class of antidepressant. Some patients are particularly intolerant to the SSRI side-effects such as sexual dysfunction, anxiety or GI side-effects, in which case switching to a different class of antidepressant would be a sensible strategy, as these side-effects appear to be specific SSRI effects.

8.61 I have found paroxetine to be a very effective drug to use, though a few patients have been unable to tolerate its side-effects. One woman, in particular, had severe night sweats. Is that common?

 Paroxetine was a market leader for SSRIs in the UK for many years and as widely used as fluoxetine. All drugs have side-effects, and the sweating you describe (in which the patient had to change the sheets and her nightdress in the middle of the night) would appear to be an unusual side-effect although well documented. Some 5% of patients will complain of some lesser but unacceptable side-effects to any of the SSRIs.

8.62 Some patients have found paroxetine rather difficult to stop taking. Why is this, and how can the problem be avoided?

 The issue of SSRI withdrawal effects is something that has been highlighted in the media, although withdrawal symptoms have been reported on stopping most antidepressants. Interestingly, withdrawal effects have supplanted the issue of suicidality and aggression with fluoxetine, and we now talk about withdrawal effects and dependency on paroxetine. Whereas withdrawal effects do undoubtedly occur, their true clinical impact is less certain. Like all powerful drugs, they should not be stopped suddenly but tailed off gradually over a matter of a few days to minimize withdrawal effects. If that fails the liquid form of paroxetine could be used and the patient could then titrate themselves down gradually over a matter of a few weeks using a syringe to measure out doses decreasing by, say, 1 mg per day.

8.63 I believe that paroxetine is no longer recommended for the treatment of depressive illness in children and adolescents. Why is that?

 New data have shown no benefit in the treatment of depression compared with placebo in those aged less than 18 years and an increase in the rate of reporting of suicidal thoughts and behaviour while on treatment. On that basis it should not be prescribed as new therapy for under-18-year-olds. For patients successfully being treated with paroxetine, completion of the course is acceptable. If the treatment is not effective it should be changed.

8.64 Is paroxetine the only drug to cease to be recommended for treatment of depression in this age group?

No, venlafaxine is also no longer recommended for the treatment of depression in children and adolescents. No other SSRI or SNRI is licensed for the treatment of children or adolescents aged less than 18 years.

8.65 Which antidepressants are licensed for the treatment of depression in children and adolescents?

No antidepressant is currently licensed for this use. Having said that, major depression is a very serious illness in children, and doctors may prescribe an antidepressant because it is the necessary treatment. They may prescribe a medicine off-licence if it is considered to be in the best interests of the patient. Non-licensed prescribing is quite widespread in psychiatric practice, as licensing requirements and clinical trials are increasingly becoming divorced from the practical realities of clinical practice. The Committee on Safety of Medicines (CSM) have set up an expert group to review the situation.

8.66 How many people receive paroxetine treatment?

Approximately 4 million prescriptions were issued for paroxetine in the UK in 2002, of which possibly 7–8000 were for patients under the age of 18. It was the market leader, with annual sales of about £100M. Venlafaxine will soon overtake it as the market leader.

8.67 What is the problem with paroxetine?

Paroxetine is a highly effective antidepressant that is used in many countries worldwide. Concern has recently been voiced over any possible association between SSRIs and suicidal behaviour, and some anecdotal evidence was screened in a TV documentary. The CSM formally reviewed this question in December 2001 and found that there was insufficient evidence to confirm a causal association between SSRIs and suicidal behaviour, though an effect in a small high-risk population could not be ruled out.

Despite the scare stories in the press, there have been no court cases where paroxetine or other antidepressants have been shown to cause or release aggression. The more obvious answer is that depression is a condition associated with a high risk of suicide. Many depressed patients are given an antidepressant and then make a suicide attempt which they would have made anyway. Alcohol, a drug well known to disinhibit people, is often taken concurrently.

LITHIUM CARBONATE

8.68 Lithium is best known as a treatment for bipolar affective disorder. Does it have a role in the treatment of depression?

Lithium is not in itself an antidepressant but does have the recognized action of 'boosting' the effects of other antidepressants when patients fail to respond to standard antidepressant treatments. As a treatment for resistant depression, there is a good case for adding a modest dose of lithium (Priadel 400 mg daily) to an antidepressant. This is likely to give a further 10–20% improvement in patients who have not responded properly and will make a few patients respond completely who have not previously responded. Lithium enhancement is probably one of the first-line treatments for resistant depression (*see Chapter 11*). The risk is that patients will develop the serotonin syndrome and become overstimulated, with anxiety, movement disorders and other strange symptoms. If this occurs the lithium should be stopped as a matter of urgency.

The other major use for lithium is as a prophylactic against relapse in both bipolar and unipolar depression, although antidepressants are probably more widely used for relapse prevention for unipolar depression (*Table 8.2*). The third use for lithium is in depressed patients who are at risk of being triggered into a manic episode by antidepressants but who need treatment because of their depression. Giving lithium at the same time as an antidepressant will reduce the risk of triggering a 'high' in these patients.

TABLE 8.2 Long-term prophylaxis against relapse of depression

Drug	Advantages	Disadvantages
Tricyclics	Tried and tested	Side-effects May precipitate mania
Modern anti-depressants	Efficacy and long-term safety data available Greater tolerability Often one tablet per day	Cost May precipitate mania
Lithium	Tried and tested formula Effective	Not antidepressant Side-effects can occur Needs monitoring of blood level Toxic to thyroid and kidney
Sodium valproate	Efficacy data emerging	Side-effects may be a problem

8.69 How does lithium work?

It works by stabilizing the cell membranes and enhancing 5HT effects on the brain. It competes with sodium for a cell membrane carrier site. It reduces the supersensitivity of dopamine receptors and increases the turnover and reuptake of noradrenaline into cells. In truth, we do not really know how lithium works.

8.70 What are its adverse effects?

 Lithium side-effects are listed in *Box 8.7*. Lithium gives rise to GI effects, tremor, feelings of muscle weakness, and polyuria and polydipsia (nephrogenic diabetes insipidus). Lithium is pharmacologically a 'bad drug' insofar as the effective dose is not far removed from the toxic dose, and it therefore needs careful blood level monitoring to maintain a plasma concentration of 0.5–0.8 mmol/L. At doses in excess of 2 mmol/L, there is the risk of serious toxicity, with neurological side-effects, coma and convulsions.

The one common serious side-effect is hypothyroidism, which can develop after a modest exposure in a significant proportion of patients (say 10%). Once it has developed, stopping lithium treatment does not necessarily result in recovery, although the first line of treatment would be to stop the lithium if clinically possible. It may be necessary to give replacement thyroxine long-term. It is therefore important to monitor thyroid function before treatment starts and at regular, say 6-monthly, reviews because hypothyroidism develops gradually and the first sign of abnormality may be an increasing level of thyroid-stimulating hormone. It may be possible to stop the process before it becomes too advanced. A different mood stabilizer might be indicated.

The other issue of concern is renal damage. Whereas polydipsia and polyuria are common occurrences, they are not in themselves dangerous. Interstitial nephritis, which could lead to renal failure, was something that caused concern in the past but is probably no more likely on lithium than without it. Again, it is usual to test for renal function every 6 months.

8.71 What precautions should be taken when prescribing and monitoring lithium treatment?

 Lithium is generally contraindicated in pregnancy because of a risk of significant harm to the fetus (mainly cardiac effects), although again the risks and benefits of treatment need to be balanced. Ideally the patient should be assessed and advised by someone with experience in these matters since overall the risks are small but the impact is great if problems occur. Lithium should be prescribed cautiously in

BOX 8.7 Main side-effects of lithium

Gastrointestinal tract

Anorexia

Nausea

Vomiting

Diarrhoea

Thirst

Incontinence

Neuromuscular changes

General muscle weakness

Ataxia

Tremor

Fasciculation and twitching

Choreoathetoid movements

Hyperactive tendon reflexes[a]

Central nervous system

Slurred speech[a]

Blurring of vision

Dizziness

Vertigo

Epileptiform seizures

Somnolence

Confusion[a]

Restlessness[a]

Stupor[a]

Coma[a]

Cardiovascular system

Hypotension

Pulse irregularities

ECG changes

Circulatory collapse

Other effects

Polyuria

Glycosuria

General fatigue[a] and lethargy[a]

Dehydration

[a] Side-effects usually associated with the toxic effects of lithium.

patients with renal impairment and advice sought from a nephrologist. Patients on long-term lithium should ideally be seen in a lithium clinic where their condition can be monitored on a routine basis. Once the patient is established on maintenance treatment, the lithium level should be checked every 6 months. A 'trough level' of the plasma concentration (12 hours after the last dose) should be measured in the morning when the morning dose is omitted. The plasma concentration should be in the range 0.5–0.8 mmol/L. Electrolytes, creatinine and thyroid function should be measured approximately every 6 months, or annually if the patient is well stabilized. Lithium should not usually interact significantly with other drugs, although there have been concerns about lithium and haloperidol causing long-term neurological damage if given together in high doses. Lithium may also cause a serotonergic syndrome when given with antidepressants.

CARBAMAZEPINE

8.72 Carbamazepine is best known to most doctors as an anti-epileptic. How does it work in the treatment of depression?

Carbamazepine is structurally similar to the tricyclic antidepressants, although pharmacologically distinct. It has complex actions. It inhibits sodium channels, and decreases the release of noradrenaline and noradrenaline activity. It interacts with GABA receptors among other actions. How this translates into an understanding of its mode of action in depressive disorders is not clear.

8.73 When is carbamazepine most likely to be useful?

As a second-line treatment when there are problems in using lithium. It may be better in rapid-cycling mood disorders when the mood swings quite rapidly from highs to lows, often several times during the day. It is also useful as an adjunctive treatment, acting as a booster to antidepressants and increasing their effectiveness in resistant cases.

8.74 Are there any serious side-effects?

The two problems to watch out for are blood dyscrasias (agranulocytosis and aplastic anaemia). The early onset of these is characterized by fevers, sore throat, a rash, bruising and mouth ulcers. The Stevens–Johnson syndrome is also a serious side-effect necessitating immediate cessation of treatment. Skin rashes are quite common.

8.75 What special precautions should be taken when prescribing and monitoring long-term treatment?

White cell and blood count and liver function tests should be carried out at the outset of treatment and after 2 weeks and then 3-monthly in order to guard against the emergence of blood dyscrasias and the Stevens–Johnson syndrome. Although this is recommended it is not a substitute for clinical vigilance, as the condition develops quite quickly and is unlikely to be picked up first on routine monitoring. Blood concentrations of the drug should be monitored to ensure it is given at the appropriate therapeutic dose. The ideal plasma concentration is in the range 7–12 mg/L, somewhat higher than the doses used in the control of epilepsy.

SODIUM VALPROATE

8.76 Sodium valproate is another drug that is known as an anticonvulsant. When is it used in psychiatry?

It is emerging as the first line treatment to replace lithium in the prophylactic treatment of bipolar mood disorders. Its position in preventing relapses in unipolar depression is less well established.

8.77 Does it have any severe adverse effects?

It is relatively free of cognitive side-effects, though alopecia and weight-gain occur frequently. The most serious side-effect is an idiosyncratic hepatotoxicity and pancreatitis.

8.78 How should treatment be monitored?

Blood levels should be checked and should be in the range 50–100 mg/L. Liver function tests should be done before treatment and at 6-monthly intervals, although raised values of LFT parameters are not uncommon and may require no specific intervention providing the prothrombin time is normal. Monitoring the overall clinical condition is the most important thing.

DIAZEPAM

8.79 Does diazepam have any antidepressant effects at all, or does it just subdue symptoms of anxiety?

Most benzodiazepine effects on depression are as a direct consequence of their action on the associated anxiety symptoms. Alprazolam is claimed to have antidepressant effects on the core symptoms of depression, but, while this may be true, they are not sufficient to justify its use as an antidepressant. The drug also causes dependency and withdrawal symptoms, and the treatment of depression may need to be continued long-term. The inappropriate use of benzodiazepines to treat depression in the past, in the mistaken belief that they were safer than antidepressants, has in my view resulted in considerable under-treatment of mood disorders, leading to chronic depression and unnecessary benzodiazepine dependence.

8.80 Where I work, patients with symptoms of depression may already have been treated with diazepam (either by their doctors or by well-meaning friends who share their pills). Presumably it is best to start treatment with an appropriate antidepressant and to try to withdraw the diazepam at a later stage. How would you tackle this problem?

Diazepam remains the most effective of all drugs in psychiatry, giving rise to substantial symptomatic relief mainly of anxiety symptoms at least in the short term. Its efficacy in long-term treatment is more controversial although it probably still remains effective, despite causing dependency and withdrawal symptoms, at least to some degree. Many patients in general practice who complain of depression also have significant or even predominant anxiety symptoms. Theoretically, patients should be treated with antidepressants and benzodiazepines and then have their benzodiazepines withdrawn gradually when the antidepressant effect becomes apparent. In my experience this rarely works, and, once patients have become dependent on the benefits of benzodiazepines, they do not improve a great deal when given antidepressants. The therapeutic dilemma then is whether to stop their benzodiazepines, which the patients like, are cheap and give some benefit, in favour of continuing with expensive modern antidepressants, which are probably not as effective as the benzodiazepines.

8.81 I found that patients who have received diazepam for their symptoms are reluctant to try antidepressants, and when they do they invariably encounter side-effects and discontinue treatment saying, 'Valium is the only thing that works for me and lets me live a normal life'. It is a very difficult problem to handle, and I wonder if you have any advice?

Benzodiazepines are unfashionable, but patients, especially those with long-term anxiety-type symptoms, do prefer benzodiazepines to antidepressants. The prevailing view is that benzodiazepines are not all that bad really, although the matter is still highly controversial.

Ultimately, each patient needs to be assessed on his or her own merits. If depressive symptoms are prevalent or if the therapeutic response is inadequate then the trial of an antidepressant should be considered. If the patients really are functioning well on a modest dose of diazepam, then there is a strong case for leaving well alone. There are still some authorities that adhere to what I take to be the outmoded dictum that 'benzodiazepines should not be prescribed long-term'. Counter to that is a strong body of general practitioner opinion that continues to prescribe long-term, presumably in the interest of their patients. The benzodiazepine debate is by no means dead, but is sadly fuelled more by prejudice than by solid scientific data.

About four million prescriptions are currently issued annually for daytime benzodiazepine anxiolytics. Alternative treatments exist; they do not cause dependency but are not without their own problems and risks.

FLUPENTIXOL

8.82 How does flupentixol work as an antidepressant?

Flupentixol is primarily an antipsychotic that acts by blockade of the D_2 receptor. Thus it has an anxiolytic action as well as an antipsychotic action by reducing dopamine activity.

At low doses, say 0.5 mg b.d., it has a paradoxical effect of blocking presynaptic dopamine autoreceptors, thereby stimulating the transmission of dopamine and acting as an antidepressant and energizer.

8.83 I sometimes use flupentixol to treat patients with mild depression coupled with anxiety. I would not use it to treat severe depression, and I think of it as a 'gentle' antidepressant. Am I right in my thinking?

Yes, it seems to be better in mild depression with prominent anxiety symptoms. It sometimes works in resistant depression where other antidepressants have failed. Whereas flupentixol often works quickly and with low side-effect problems, it does have the small risk of causing tardive dyskinesia and other extrapyramidal symptoms on occasions.

ANTIPSYCHOTICS

8.84 Do some of the newer antipsychotic drugs have mood-elevating properties?

There is no direct evidence of antidepressant activity by themselves. They would appear to be sedative and anxiolytic in the same way that traditional antipsychotics are. There is some evidence that olanzapine given in conjunction with antidepressants causes an enhanced antidepressant effect. Antipsychotics can be used for long-term prophylaxis, especially olanzapine.

8.85 Depression and schizophrenia may coexist. How would you treat this combination?

Depression may coexist with schizophrenia as one of the core symptoms of schizophrenia, in which case the correct treatment would be to manage the schizophrenic illness with full doses of antipsychotic drugs. Conversely, depression may be a function of either drug side-effects of the treatment for the schizophrenic illness or for psychological reasons associated with the illness. For example, as insight returns, patients may for very valid reasons be upset at the implications of having a long-term serious mental illness. Patients may suffer not so much depression but a 'lack of mood' as a function of the 'negative symptoms of schizophrenia'. Depression is also a common condition and may coexist independently of the schizophrenic illness. Bearing in mind what a horrible condition schizophrenia is, I think an early trial of antidepressant medication is indicated if the patient is depressed, since whatever the reason it may help alleviate at least some of the symptoms that the patients have.

THYROXINE

8.86 Does thyroxine have any mood-elevating properties?

Hypothyroidism is a well-known cause of tiredness and low mood, and correcting the condition with thyroxine is a gratifying therapeutic endeavour. Thyroxine by itself is not an antidepressant drug in depressive illnesses. Thyroxine is a potent adjunct treatment given in low doses to enhance the therapeutic effects of antidepressants in cases of resistant depression. Lithium, which is used in the control of mood disorders, can in some patients cause an insidious hypothyroidism, in which case of course this should be treated with thyroxine as well as by adjusting and potentially stopping lithium treatment. Hyperthyroidism and hypothyroidism can both give rise to symptoms that mimic mood disorders.

8.87 When is thyroxine used in the treatment of depression?

Thyroxine is added to an antidepressant in the treatment of resistant depression. The dose is 20–50 micrograms of tri-iodothyronine. Thyroid functioning needs to be monitored. It is also used in 'subclinical hypothyroidism', although this condition is more controversial as an entity which may be a function of a mood disorder. Hypothalamic instability may be associated with suicidal behaviour and associated depression, and so it is worth treating hypothyroidism in depressed patients vigorously.

ELECTROCONVULSIVE THERAPY (ECT)

8.88 How does ECT work in the treatment of depression?

ECT down-regulates beta-receptors and enhances central neurotransmission in a manner similar to antidepressants. It also affects GABA-B receptors and central muscarinic receptors, which may be the mechanism of the post-therapy memory deficits. The precise mode of action of ECT remains a matter of conjecture, but the benefits as the most effective treatment for severe depression are not in doubt.

8.89 Is ECT still used, and if so on whom?

ECT is primarily used for the treatment of severe depression that is not responsive to antidepressants. It is also used for patients who are in depressive stupors and unable to eat and drink, and is particularly indicated in patients with depressive delusions. It can also be used in acute mania and psychosis. It is the most effective treatment for severe depression, and probably the safest, and is generally under-used.

The superiority of ECT over antidepressants is most pronounced in the severely ill patient, and it is mainly kept in reserve as a treatment of last resort. In the milder cases the benefit is less marked, and treatment with antidepressants is probably more acceptable.

8.90 How is ECT administered, and do patients find it upsetting and painful or unpleasant?

Prior to the procedure, patients have the treatment explained to them. They should be reassured of its benefits. The treatment itself is administered after an anaesthetic and muscle relaxant has been administered. A current of about 150 millicoulombs is passed either bilaterally between the patient's temples or unilaterally between the frontal cortex and the mastoid bone on the non-dominant hemisphere. After the current has passed, the patient usually exhibits some minor twitching of the toes. The patient wakes up a few minutes later, with no memory of the actual treatment and remains dazed for an hour or so. Within an hour or so the patient makes a full recovery and can resume normal activities a few hours later and even go to work. The worst side-effect is a memory problem around the time of the treatment – this is usually not severe and tends to recover with time. The major problem is one of anxiety and prejudice about the procedure, rather than the procedure itself.

8.91 What is the difference between unilateral and bilateral ECT?

Bilateral ECT may be more effective. Unilateral ECT given to the non-dominant hemisphere appears to cause fewer memory problems.

8.92 What are the side-effects of ECT, and do these eventually limit its use?

The most troublesome side-effect is memory loss. Patients complain of strange gaps in their memory, especially for people's names and details of events. It is maximal around the time of treatment and improves over the following weeks and months. This troublesome side-effect is not universal, and needs to be balanced against the harmful effects of severe, untreated depression and prolonged hospitalization. Side-effects can be minimized by giving unilateral ECT to the non-dominant hemisphere. In some cases if memory loss becomes troublesome, the course of ECT may be terminated prematurely. Otherwise, side-effects are rare and limited mainly to the hazard of anaesthetic or to musculoskeletal problems, both of which are extremely rare.

8.93 Do patients have to consent to ECT?

Patients have to consent to ECT and sign a consent form. There are interesting issues around consent for people who are severely depressed. The patient has to be able to give a 'valid consent'. If patients are not willing or able to give consent, then ECT can be administered if the patient is detained under Section 3 of the Mental Health Act (a treatment order). A 'second-opinion doctor' from the Mental Health Act Commission is then required to certify that the treatment is appropriate, in which case treatment can proceed without the patient's consent. In exceptional circumstances where a patient is severely suicidal or in a stupor, ECT can be given as an emergency procedure to save a patient's life without consent. There are problems with patients who, because of their illness, are unable to consent although they do not refuse. For example, they may be in a depressive stupor and unable to communicate. In such cases they should be treated under the Mental Health Act. (*See also Chapter 13.*)

8.94 Do patients have to consent to each individual treatment?

Patients have to sign a consent form for the whole course of ECT. This should only happen after all the options available as alternatives to ECT have been discussed. The patient can always withdraw consent at any time, and the patient can refuse treatment even when some treatments have already been administered. Things have moved on a great deal from the days of *One Flew Over the Cuckoo's Nest*. The rights and safeguards of patients are now paramount.

8.95 Does consent still have to be sought when a patient is in hospital under a section of the Mental Health Act?

If patients are detained under the Mental Health Act, they have to be able and willing to consent to the treatment for it to proceed. Just because they are sectioned does not mean they are unable to consent or do not have to consent. If they are unable or unwilling to consent then compulsory treatment can be given if a 'second opinion doctor' on behalf of the Mental Health Act Commission certifies that the treatment is appropriate (you don't have to say it is the best treatment – only that it is appropriate).

8.96 How dangerous is ECT?

The danger of ECT is essentially that of the anaesthetic. There are about two deaths per hundred thousand treatments.

8.97 What is RTMS and how does it work?

Repetitive transcranial magnetic stimulation (RTMS) is a treatment in which the brain is stimulated using a hand-held magnetic coil focused onto selective brain regions. The patient remains awake during the treatment without needing an anaesthetic. The electromagnetic stimulation activates particularly the dorsolateral prefrontal cortex, increasing the activity in this area. Patients find the treatment less stigmatizing and safer than ECT. A typical treatment course involves daily brief outpatient sessions over 2–3 weeks. The treatment is still being evaluated, but it appears to be about as effective as antidepressants and less effective than ECT. It is still an experimental procedure.

8.98 What advantages does it offer over traditional ECT?

It does not require an anaesthetic, it is less stigmatizing with less drama attached to it. It is seen as more modern and acceptable. It appears to be low on side-effects. There is less memory impairment.

PATIENT QUESTIONS

8.99   What types of treatment are available for depression?

There are two main types of treatment available: medication and psychological or 'talking' treatments. Medication in the form of antidepressants is probably the most effective treatment for moderate to severe depression. It works in most patients within a few weeks and gives reasonable relief of symptoms in most patients. Antidepressants make people feel better. Psychological treatments help people understand the roots of their symptoms and how their lifestyle and relationships have led to them feeling depressed. It helps people deal with the consequences of depression. Patients often want to talk about their symptoms. Talking treatments tend to take longer to work. They are often seen as more appropriate for milder depressions, especially those caused by lifestyle and relationship problems. Medication and psychological treatments in combination may well be the best option if available. Cognitive behaviour therapy (CBT) is a psychological treatment that helps people learn to do things and control their thoughts to make them feel better.

There are other treatments such as hypnosis and homeopathic remedies, social treatments, exercise and all manner of alternative approaches including St John's Wort. These tend to be more appropriate for the milder forms of depression. Hospital admission and even ECT may on rare occasions be needed for the most severe forms where the depression may be life threatening or cause major problems for the individual. There is a broad range of treatment options available.

8.100   Will I become dependent on antidepressants?

Antidepressants are not addictive in the way that illicit drugs, alcohol or tranquillizers can be. Most patients take antidepressants for a brief period of time and then gradually stop taking them without any problems. Some patients develop mild withdrawal symptoms if they stop the antidepressant suddenly, and so patients are advised to cut down antidepressants gradually over a matter of weeks rather than stopping abruptly. Even then, withdrawal symptoms don't always occur, and if they do they tend to be relatively mild and usually last only a few days, even if the antidepressants are stopped suddenly. Some patients become reliant upon antidepressants for keeping their symptoms under control. When they stop their medication they relapse. On that basis it becomes a choice of whether the benefits of staying on medication outweigh the disadvantages or whether the patients prefer to put up with their symptoms rather than take medication. Some patients may try alternative treatments rather than taking antidepressants long-term. This becomes a value judgement really for the patient to make in conjunction with their doctor, based on sound information from the doctor and informed choice by the patient.

 PATIENT QUESTIONS

8.101 Will it be difficult stopping antidepressant therapy?

The vast majority of patients stop antidepressant treatment, without seeking the advice of their doctors, simply because they want to. In doing so they have no problems at all. Most doctors spend a lot of time persuading patients to carry on taking antidepressants rather than persuading patients to stop them. Most patients have no trouble stopping antidepressants at all. If they are stopped suddenly, then some patients develop mild withdrawal symptoms lasting a day or two and these are generally tolerable. The symptoms may include dizziness, 'electric shock' feelings, anxiety and agitation, insomnia, flu-like symptoms, diarrhoea, nausea, tingling feelings and mood swings. If there are any problems, the antidepressant should be cut down over a number of days, either by reducing the dose gradually, or taking the tablets on alternate days, then every third day.

8.102 Do I have to inform the DVLA that I am taking antidepressants?

Straightforward anxiety and depression does not need to be notified to the DVLA. If there are problems relating to memory, agitation or suicidal thinking, then this needs to be notified. If the condition may make the driver dangerous, this must be notified, and the DVLA may then make enquiries to decide whether the licence should be withdrawn. There is no obligation to notify the DVLA if you are taking antidepressants, providing you are aware that all medication can impair alertness, concentration and driving performance especially within the first month of starting medication or increasing the dose. If you experience any problems then you should not drive. Sedative antidepressants are more likely to cause drowsiness, and antidepressants can interact with other drugs and tranquillizers as well as alcohol. In general, drivers with depression are safer when well and on regular antidepressant medication than when ill. If in doubt about your fitness to drive you should not drive and should notify the DVLA. It is the illness and the general condition that you suffer from that is the most important thing rather than the medication that you are taking.

8.103 Why do I have to go on taking tablets once I feel better?

Not everyone has to continue on tablets once they feel better. If you have had a severe depression, and were to stop taking the tablets, there is a risk that you will slip back and become depressed again. The longer you take the tablets the less the risk becomes, and after 6 months of feeling well, the risks of becoming depressed again when you stop the tablets are low, and so we generally recommend taking tablets for 6 months after you feel better to avoid relapsing too soon.

8.104 Should my child stop taking Seroxat immediately?

No. If your child is benefiting, it may well be appropriate to continue with the drug. If it is decided to stop the drug, it is important that it be tailed off gradually to avoid discontinuation or withdrawal symptoms. It is best to discuss this with your GP or psychiatrist.

Treatment of depression – psychological therapies

9

9.1 How widely available are psychological therapies?

Psychological therapies, which primarily involve talking rather than taking medication, are becoming increasingly popular in the UK. Patients are increasingly of the belief that talking about their problem will make it go away – though doing this is not necessarily the same as a specific therapy. Nevertheless about half of GP practices now have in-house therapists. These are for the most part counsellors. There will be access to community psychiatric nurses (CPNs) who will have a broader mental-health background, and some will have specific cognitive behavioural therapy (CBT) training. Cognitive behavioural therapists tend to be in shorter supply. In the UK we are still a long way behind the USA in the acceptability and availability of therapists.

Patients may be confused about different disciplines and styles of therapy ranging from counselling to analytically based therapy and the more structured CBT. There is an increasing emphasis on brief focused therapy. Family therapy and marital therapy as well as anger management therapy are being advocated. An expanding number of different types of therapy are becoming available, including hypnotherapy, but there is still a wide variation in what is available throughout the UK and between countries. Therapy can often be accessed through professional organizations, and if patients have an alcohol or drug problem then it is often easier to access specialist therapists through the substance misuse service than to go through the conventional psychiatric route. There is often a substantial delay in accessing more structured therapy such as CBT. This is particularly problematic when the evidence is that early intervention is so much more effective than delaying treatment. Detailed psychoanalytic therapy may be almost unavailable outside of the major centres, and, even if it is available, the waiting time for treatment may be very long. For ready access to a skilled therapist, patients may often find it appropriate to pay for their treatment if they can afford to do so.

COUNSELLING

9.2 What is counselling?

Counselling is a broad term for a psychotherapeutic treatment in which patients are encouraged to understand themselves and their problems, to give them a greater sense of control over their lives and consequently to improve their self-esteem. In counselling, patients are encouraged to work out their own solutions to their problems and to try and understand how their problems have arisen, possibly in relation to past experiences. Counselling is very much in the 'here and now' and dealing with conscious as opposed to unconscious mental processes. More-formal psychotherapy deals more with unconscious matters and the relationship between the therapist and the patient. Cognitive behavioural therapy looks more at behaviours and feelings and how to deal with them. Counselling is a more superficial treatment, encouraging patients to clarify their problems and to find new solutions to things that can be changed and to find ways of dealing with problems that cannot be altered.

9.3 How is talking to someone about a problem likely to help?

Counselling can help patients cope with a crisis, reflect on the situation and move on. Therapy can help people deal with a crisis, can provide support and help them restructure their thinking. It can help patients by providing a non-judgemental ready ear so that they can themselves think their way through their situation. Counsellors should avoid giving direct advice but should encourage patients to reflect on a situation and develop coping strategies. The therapist should not be too challenging and analytical lest rapid confrontation increase stresses. Therapists should aim to increase patients' understanding of themselves and their problems. Often a problem aired and shared is a problem halved. In addition, specific coping strategies can be discussed such as anxiety management or even simple problem solving and maybe the rudiments of CBT. Patients benefit from not feeling alone and having a focus to work on.

9.4 How can a person find a counsellor and be confident that he or she is properly trained?

Many GP practices now have counsellors attached to them. The GP should be able to recommend one to a patient and in turn should be satisfied that the counsellor is appropriately trained or recognized by a professional body. In addition, personal qualities of maturity and insight and empathy may be as important as formal training. The GP may have established a working relationship with several counsellors who can be recommended, or whom he or she has got to know by personal recommendation. Sadly, although there are many reputable bodies that are attempting to register counsellors, there is still not a uniform standard.

9.5 How can a GP judge which counsellors to recommend?

They should have undergone a recognized training and be registered with an accredited professional body. Unfortunately there are no universally accepted standards yet. The counsellor should be interviewed, ideally not only by the GP but also by another counsellor as well, to assess not only the quality of the training, but also the personal qualities of the counsellor – qualities such as maturity, empathy, patience and understanding are important. Finally, if a candidate looks promising, he or she can be offered a trial period of referrals to see how the patients react. Basically if the counsellor has had an adequate training, then it is really the personal qualities that count.

9.6 Can counselling be combined with antidepressant therapy?

Most certainly, yes. Antidepressants are effective at relieving symptoms; counselling deals with helping people to understand how they have found themselves in particular situations and how relationships and thought processes have resulted in their symptoms. Counselling may alter behaviour, actions and thoughts but not necessarily symptoms. Antidepressants tend not to work if the symptoms are mild, and counselling tends not to work if the symptoms are severe and dominate the patient's thinking. Sometimes patients need to have their symptoms relieved before they can concentrate on the work necessary for counselling.

9.7 Are some forms of counselling more appropriate to specific situations?

Counsellors should be flexible and adapt their approach to the situation. On the other hand, some counsellors may not have the breadth of clinical experience to deal with all sorts of problems. A specific example would be drug counselling, where a different approach is needed from that for, say, a bereavement. The ability to work with individuals in a particular situation and to establish credibility with them is important. Marriage guidance takes particular skills, especially the ability to deal with couples. Psychosexual counselling, again, requires a knowledge of particular behavioural therapy techniques (e.g. Masters and Johnson), while other counsellors specialize in HIV, and also bereavement therapies. Thus although the root principles remain the same, and many counsellors have experience in more than one area, different types of problems require specific approaches and you are unlikely to find a counsellor who feels comfortable and can be effective in all areas.

9.8 What sort of supervision do counsellors have?

Counsellors should be supervised by an experienced therapist or counsellor to help them to see potential difficulties which are easier to observe from outside than from within a therapeutic situation. For example a patient may make unreasonable demands upon the counsellor who would like to help but fails to see the dangers of becoming over-involved with the patient. It is sometimes difficult to see, from within the therapeutic relationship, the direction in which the situation is moving, and outside advice helps to keep matters on track. A supervisor should be able to spot the danger signs and try to avert them. The GP should also be able to supervise a counsellor and be available as a backstop in case the situation deteriorates or the patient makes demands in excess of what the counsellor can fulfil, or if the clinical situation demonstrates and requires medication or specialist referral. The GP should be prepared to maintain a dialogue with the counsellor and to be available if problems occur.

9.9 What is person-centred counselling?

This is a non-directive form of therapy described by Carl Rogers, who stated that the most important qualities of a therapist were empathy, warmth and understanding. The therapy is client-centred and the client is always in control of what is discussed. The counsellor helps the client to work out better ways of dealing with problems, by listening, answering questions and trying to understand, and then reflecting back, for example by rephrasing what the client has said in a more sympathetic and understanding way. If a client says that there is a problem in dealing with his or her boss, the therapist might respond with the question, 'Why do you think you have troubles dealing with your boss?', which would require the client to explore the issue further. No direct advice or interpretation is given, and the aim of the counselling is to get clients to change their perceptions and attitudes at the end of therapy. In the example used here, the client would understand better the relationship with his or her boss, and the emotional impact of the difficulty would be understood and reduced.

PSYCHOTHERAPY

9.10 How does psychotherapy differ from counselling?

The main difference is in the degree to which the 'unconscious' feelings are explored. In counselling, work is really done in the 'here and now'. In psychoanalytic therapy, the patient not only discusses the problems but tries to make a link to how these problems have emerged as a function of past life experiences, often in childhood and previous relationships (see Case study 9.1). These relationships are then explored within the context of the psychotherapeutic relationship. Psychotherapy deals with helping the patient to understand how they are motivated by unconscious anxieties. Therapy is usually deeper and lasts longer than counselling. Psychotherapy is often founded on disciplines such as theories of Freud or Jung and has a much more structured framework within which to work than counselling.

CASE STUDY 9.1 A PSYCHOTHERAPEUTIC INTERPRETATION
After a number of therapeutic sessions, the patient becomes rather hostile and rejecting of the therapist and expresses the belief that the therapist is not taking him seriously. The interpretation is that the patient is re-enacting his relationship with his mother, whom he felt did not take him seriously. He also feels that other important people in his life did not take him seriously, causing difficulties in his relationships. An interpretation of what has happened in the relationship between the patient and therapist provides an explanation of how the patient projects his anxieties about his early experiences into his current life.

9.11 What forms of psychotherapy are available, and how does someone choose the right one?

This is a difficult question, and the answer depends on many factors. Partly it depends on personal preference and personal recommendation as well as what is available locally. Group therapies are not only cost-effective in terms of one therapist seeing many clients, but probably the treatment of choice when it comes to alcohol difficulties or domestic violence. Group pressure is important when confronting individuals over their problems in a way that an individual therapist may not be able to do so ('it takes one to know one'). Patients often benefit from being involved with other fellow sufferers, and group dynamics enable the re-enactment of subconscious emotions and behaviours, which can express themselves through the group in a way that they cannot with an individual therapist. Individual therapy is more appropriate for people who have trouble expressing themselves verbally. Family therapy is of course important where the problem is part of a family interaction rather than a problem of an individual.

If there is any doubt about the appropriate way to proceed then the opinion of a specialist should be sought, or your local counsellor could have exploratory sessions to see which way things should progress. Failing that you could seek an opinion from a local consultant psychotherapist to decide on how appropriate therapy is for the individual and what the most appropriate therapy is. This process may take time but may reap benefits in the long run. Psychotherapy should not be embarked upon lightly. It is hard work and not an easy option.

Another consideration is that not all patients are appropriate to undergo psychotherapy, and before embarking upon the lengthy road it may be more appropriate to test motivation and ability to work and to undergo 'change' as opposed to simply turning up and talking and not using the therapy in a constructive way. It may be appropriate to engage patients in a relatively straightforward approach, such as relaxation therapy, for a limited period of time in order to assess their suitability for more structured longer-term work, their ability to turn up regularly and their commitment to work in a structured way. A lot of resources are wasted on patients who drop out of therapy after one or two sessions because they are unable to make the commitment to working on their problem, or were not aware of what was involved.

9.12 Have all psychotherapists undergone therapy themselves?

Psychotherapists should have undergone some form of training therapy themselves. This is because psychotherapy is very much a 'process', and the best way to learn the process is through going through the procedure yourself to understand it rather than through didactic teaching. Part of the training involves treating clients under supervision, but an essential part is having the experience yourself.

One important issue is how to deal with your own feelings about the patient (counter-transference). It is important to know when your experiences and gut feelings and emotional interaction with the patient result from the patient's effect upon you and to what degree your feelings and experiences result from your personal prejudices. For example, is the patient making unreasonable demands on you, or does your own view of the world lead you to think that people make unreasonable demands on you? Once therapists are qualified, they then need to continue and be supervised with regular sessions with the supervisor to help them deal with personal difficulties that arise as a result of the therapy and their interaction with the client.

9.13 What is brief focal psychotherapy, and what are its advantages in the general-practice setting?

This therapy is thought to be the most appropriate form of psychotherapy for use in general practice. It is more symptom oriented than problem oriented and is provided in a limited number of sessions. Ultimately it may be as effective for a given problem as longer therapies, and it is certainly cheaper in time and money. The disadvantage is that it may not deal with the underlying problem causing the distress.

It is a relatively simple form of treatment that does not work on a deep psychoanalytical level, and should be suitable for a sympathetic GP or practice nurse with appropriate training to apply. It offers a simple framework in which patients are asked to explore their problems, and they do the work in finding solutions themselves. The therapist's role is to ask an appropriate question when an issue has been defined.

9.14 What is Gestalt therapy?

This therapy was developed in the 1940s in America. It deals mainly with the 'here and now'. It concentrates on the whole person and their relationship with the physical world. It examines issues such as how the client expresses emotion through physical posture. It encourages patients to let their feelings out, by, for example, releasing aggression through punching pillows, rather than repressing them. It examines how people express their feelings.

TRANSACTIONAL ANALYSIS (TA)

9.15 What is TA?

The concept comes from the book *Games People Play*, by Eric Berne. The life of the client is analysed in terms of how the roles that develop in childhood are played out in adult life. Behaviours are analysed in terms of the child, adult and parent within and how that results in the way that people react with others in their relationships.

9.16 How is it helpful?

It helps clients understand where their attitudes and feelings and behaviours come from in a rather simple and populist way. It is not as threatening as a full analysis and can be used for example in organizational settings to understand people who do not necessarily see themselves as sick or as patients but as part of an organization.

9.17 Who might benefit?

It is a relatively straightforward therapy for intelligent and verbal individuals who are not necessarily unwell or patients. It can be useful in analysing behaviours in organizations and how, for example, people interact at work or in their families.

COGNITIVE AND ANALYTICAL THERAPY (CAT)

9.18 What is CAT?

It is a short-term focused treatment, developed by Anthony Ryle, using psychoanalytical principles that can overlap with CBT. It examines feelings related to behaviours as well as the behaviours themselves. For example, if a specific situation causes anxiety, an analysis of the feeling of anxiety may help to understand its origins. By dealing with the original conflict through explanation, the current anxieties and consequent problematic behaviour patterns can be understood and possibly resolved.

9.19 How does CAT work in the treatment of depression?

As people come to understand their unconscious thoughts and feelings, their insight increases and their feelings of depression and distress are thereby reduced.

9.20 Is CAT any more or less effective than antidepressant drugs in minor depression?

I'm not sure that a direct comparison is appropriate. Firstly drugs are not necessarily effective in minor depression. Drugs tend to improve symptoms, whereas therapy helps patients understand their symptoms and problems and thereby, it is hoped, feel better. Therefore therapy and drugs have a different treatment outcome and are not directly comparable. Hence the debate over therapy versus drugs is unhelpful.

9.21 Can CAT be used in combination with antidepressant drugs, and is the combination more effective than either drugs or CAT alone?

There was a view, which essentially came from classical psychoanalysis, that patients needed to have symptoms in order to drive change, and that if symptoms were removed by medication then the driving force for change was removed. Whereas this view may have an intellectual consistency, it does not appear to be borne out in practical therapeutic situations. The alternative view is that medication reduces symptoms to a degree where therapy can work. In general, therapy works better for people whose conditions are not dominated by symptoms. Therapy does not work with people who are severely depressed. In an ideal world patients should be offered the benefits of both treatments providing they are helpful. A lot depends on what the therapeutic goal is: symptom relief, improved function, or understanding.

9.22 Is CAT alone effective in the treatment of major depression?

Probably not. It may be of some benefit in the treatment of moderate depression but not in depression when it is severe. CAT is probably more effective in helping people understand why and how they feel that way and how they cope with difficulties in real life rather than in symptom relief.

9.23 Is CAT effective in the treatment of recurrent depression?

It may be effective if the depression is a result of long-standing problems in relationships that then cause recurrent depressive symptoms.

9.24 How does treatment with CAT compare with conventional antidepressant treatment on a cost basis?

The hope is that therapy can in some way correct the underlying defect that causes depression and therefore make longer-term treatment with antidepressants unnecessary. Unfortunately this is not really borne out in reality. Simple cost comparisons are difficult. You have to take into account not only the therapist's time but also the costs of the building and the time of the patient. You need to pay for the administrators who run the service, and so therapy gets expensive. To calculate the drug costs, one has to decide how much the medication actually helps the patient or whether there is a placebo response. Also the outcomes are more variable.

COGNITIVE BEHAVIOUR THERAPY (CBT)

9.25 What is CBT?

CBT is a general approach to psychological and psychiatric problems that developed over the last fifty years or so, initially based on learning theory. The basic behavioural view is that if you do things that ordinarily give you pleasure then with time your depression will lift. The cognitive model deals with changing thoughts from unhelpful ones such as 'there is no solution' to problem solving and finding solutions. Thus through changing thinking and behaviour, mood can be improved. The general approach begins with an assessment of the patient's problems in terms of what they are actually doing and what they are thinking while they are doing it. Patients can keep records of their activities, and their thoughts and mood can be examined. Ways are then developed to explore these thoughts to help patients arrive at more helpful ways of looking at the world. Behaviours and thoughts that are frequently repeated and quantifiable are easier to change than rare and nebulous distress such as existential crises. Phobias, for example, are often treated successfully.

An example of the vicious spiral of negative thinking that maintains depression is given in *Figure 9.1*. CBT aims to break this spiral. The principles of CBT are outlined in *Box 9.1*. *Figure 9.2* gives an example of entries from a diary in which a patient records thoughts and feelings.

9.26 How does it work in the treatment of depression?

It provides a structured framework for dealing with depressive problems. Patients are encouraged to look at their problems in a positive way and, with the help of a therapist, seek practical solutions in structured ways (*see Case study 9.2*). They analyse a situation to avoid the all-or-nothing view of catastrophic thinking. They tackle small problems in a positive way and thereby learn to generalize this approach to larger problems. As small problems get solved, bigger ones become more accessible.

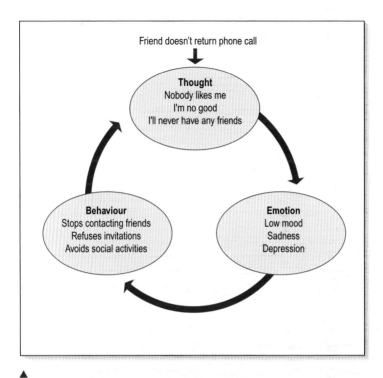

Fig. 9.1 An example of the vicious spiral of negative thinking that maintains depression.

CASE STUDY 9.2 AN EXAMPLE OF CBT FOR DEPRESSION

A depressed woman has a negative view of life and herself. Her partner has recently left her. The therapist helps her to look at her positive attributes: her job, her friends and success in other aspects of living. The issue is raised that the partner may be not have been right for her and that the relationship was not as ideal as she suggests. The break-up may not have been her fault as she believes. The therapist points out that, as a result of her depression, she has stopped working, seeing friends and exercising – all activities with antidepressant properties. As she resumes these pleasurable activities and avoids a preoccupation with self-doubt, the depression begins to lift.

9.27 Is CBT more or less effective than antidepressant drugs in minor depression?

Again there is no real comparison between the outcomes in the two. Antidepressants are not much more effective than placebo in minor

BOX 9.1 Principles of CBT

- Analysis of problem – focusing on how thinking affects emotions and behaviour
- The antecedents – behaviour, beliefs and consequences
- A formulation of the problem that can be tested in daily life
- Daily monitoring of thoughts and behaviour with a personal diary to plot progress
- Patients describe their thoughts associated with their symptoms in the treatment session
- Homework – patients have tasks to complete: for example to approach situations that provoke anxiety and to do it repeatedly whilst practising anxiety reduction, changing thoughts and thinking rationally about the situation, and recording progress and thinking
- Reading standard self-help books, such as *Living with Fear* by Isaac Marks, to understand the underlying condition

depression. CBT may well give superior results providing the patient persists with the treatment. The advantage of CBT is that it is one of the psychological therapies that lends itself to easy outcome measurement and is of proven benefit in a variety of conditions. Both antidepressants and CBT are of proven benefit in the treatment of depression.

9.28 How do you help people who are depressed and stuck because of their behaviour patterns?

This is the classic situation addressed by CBT. Because patients are depressed they do depressive things and thereby do not participate in mood-enhancing behaviour that will lead them out of depression. A classic example is that depressed people stop socializing and therefore become withdrawn and avoid the pleasurable activities and interactions with others, and this worsens their depression. Patients should be encouraged to look at simple CBT techniques to deal with their depressive thoughts and behaviours. By doing pleasurable activities, their mood will at least be temporarily improved, leading to the ability to do more complex mood-enhancing behaviours.

For example, I try to encourage my patients to go to the cinema once a week or to ring up an old friend and arrange a meeting maybe three times a week, just so that they do not become too isolated and spend too much time sitting alone at home, brooding. A more complicated programme might involve drawing up a list of simple mood-enhancing activities which can then be dealt with on a regular basis in small steps. This will start with

Date	Situation Actual event or stream of thoughts/memories	Feelings Rate 0–100	Negative thoughts Rate belief in thought 0–100	Rational answers Consider: evidence, alternatives, effects of negative thinking, thinking errors	Re-rate Negative thoughts and feelings
8 Dec	Dropped mug of coffee	Upset 80%	Things never go right for me 85% I'm stupid to feel this way 90%	I'm feeling depressed so it's hard to cope and even little things upset me. It won't go on forever, plenty of things have worked out in the past. It's not stupid to feel bad, and it doesn't mean that I'm stupid	Upset 50% Things never go right 60% I'm stupid 50%
9 Dec	Didn't get an interview for a job I applied for a month ago	Depressed 90%	They think I'm no good 100% I'm a failure 95% I'll never get another job 95%	Lots of people applied for that job. It was very popular. Just because I didn't get an interview doesn't mean I'll never get a job (I'm over-generalising and predicting the future when I think that). I've been pretty good at getting jobs in the past. To be honest, I knew it was a long shot when I applied but I felt OK then. My skills didn't really fit the job description. Telling myself I'm a failure doesn't help me in getting a job.	Depressed 40% They think I'm no good 40% I'm a failure 60% I'll never get another job 40%

Fig. 9.2 Challenging negative thoughts with a thought diary.

simple activities at first, such as getting up and getting dressed by a certain time in the day, and possibly going out to look at shops or to go to a museum or whatever it is the patient actually enjoys doing – possibly playing a round of golf or having a hair-do (depending upon gender and interest). These are activities that a CPN can encourage a patient to take on in small and increasing steps, thereby unravelling the pattern of depressive behaviours.

9.29 Can CBT be used in combination with antidepressant drugs, and is a combination more effective than either drugs or CBT alone?

CBT does not really work well if patients are very depressed. Antidepressants can lift the mood to enable patients to do the more detailed work to create longer-term change and to prevent relapse. The best approach is to treat the symptoms first with an antidepressant and then, when the symptoms are more under control, to embark upon a programme of CBT. The referral to the therapist can be made while the antidepressants are beginning to work.

9.30 Does CBT have a role to play in the treatment of bipolar disorder and recurrent depression?

To a small degree it may help avoid the stresses and strains of mood disorders and enable patients to control the worst of their mood swings. It enables parents to develop coping strategies and aids compliance with medication. It may reduce relapse rates.

HYPNOTHERAPY

9.31 What is hypnotherapy, and how does it differ from other forms of psychotherapy?

Hypnotherapy is a form of treatment that involves a state of hypnosis. Hypnosis is a state of deep suggestibility when the patient is able to focus directly on the therapist to the exclusion of other extraneous distractions. In this state of heightened suggestibility and reduced defences, the therapist can then explore hidden fears, anxieties and conflicts and importantly place post-hypnotic suggestions. The treatment is particularly useful in reducing anxiety. It can help by overcoming phobias initially in the imagination but then in real life. It can help patients to give up smoking, for example – they will experience a cigarette as tasting bad after post-hypnotic suggestion.

Hypnosis is a technique that places the patient in a profound state of relaxation at one level but otherwise in a heightened state of concentration on the therapist, in order for him or her to become suggestible at a subliminal level. It is not possible to make patients do things they do not want to do, but it helps them to achieve certain psychological goals if they wish them to happen. For example, the therapist can explore sexual feelings to which the patient might ordinarily be too anxious to admit. It uses techniques of dissociation and was therefore originally used in the treatment of hysteria. Patients vary in their suggestibility and hence in the degree to which hypnosis may be of help.

9.32 Is hypnotherapy particularly useful in certain conditions?

It is useful for anxiety, phobias and addictions. Originally, in the 19th century, hypnosis was used as a treatment for hysteria, but this is a very rare and dangerous condition to diagnose (because the diagnosis may be wrong). Because it works via suggestion at a subliminal level, hypnosis is useful for anxiety states when patients can relax themselves using a technique very similar to standard relaxation techniques and progressive muscular relaxation. It helps patients relive and re-enact repressed trauma in a controlled way, thus enabling a resolution of conflicts and anxieties that would be too stressful to deal with if the patient were not hypnotized. It can be used as a form of desensitization in the imagination for phobic patients, who can approach their feared objects in a relaxed disassociated state. In all these conditions, hypnosis works in a similar fashion to non-hypnotic techniques for dealing with the problem, but because of the additive effect of suggestion and relaxation, progress can be faster and more profound than without hypnosis. It is a more mechanical treatment than conventional therapy, because the treatment does more of the work in putting suggestions to the patient rather than the patient's doing the exploratory work.

Hypnosis is of particular value in pain management, either in acute situations such as in a dental treatment, or for chronic pain where patients can alter their focus of attention and disassociate from the pain, possibly by some functional change in the nervous system. In the treatment of smoking addiction and eating disorders, hypnosis can have an additive effect on the patient's own resolve by the power of suggestion. However, there are also problems with hypnosis. Despite dramatic demonstrations of its power and popularity among its protagonists, demonstrating clinical efficacy remains a problem. Some patients develop a strong attachment to their therapist, and only a limited proportion of patients are good subjects for hypnosis.

9.33 Patients tend to worry about being hypnotized as part of their treatment and feel they might be influenced against their wishes in some way. Can people be hypnotized against their will or forced to do anything they do not want to do?

Patients vary in their ability to be hypnotic subjects. Some very suggestible people can be hypnotized in a small way against their will, but not to any deep level. Usually subjects are willing participants, and hypnosis only enables them to do what they really want to. Hypnotherapy is a more rapid way to reach a state of communication between therapist and patient but not a way for the therapist to take over control. The therapist cannot make patients do things that they would not wish to do.

9.34 Can people hypnotize themselves and, if so, is this a useful technique?

One of the most helpful aspects of hypnosis is learning how to 'self hypnotize'. Having learnt relaxation and distraction and other techniques in the hypnotic session, patients can then induce a hypnotic state at times of tranquillity and can do their homework, once or twice a day, thus enhancing the benefit of treatment substantially. Hypnosis, as in so many other therapies, works best if the patient then takes control of his or her own situation, rather than being a passive recipient of treatment. Homework and repeated self-hypnosis will increase the power and efficacy of the treatment. The more you practise, the better you get.

PSYCHOANALYSIS

9.35 What is psychoanalysis?

This is a system of understanding the functioning of the mind developed by Freud and his contemporaries at the end of the 19th century. It is distinct from psychotherapy in that it does not specifically look at treatment but is more a system for understanding mental function. A basic principle is related to the issue that what we do and feel results from forces and processes that we are not necessarily aware of – the unconscious mind. It draws relationships between past experiences and the present. It pays particular attention to dreams as a way of understanding unconscious thoughts. Classical psychoanalysis involves a therapist seeing a patient up to five times a week for fifty-minute sessions over a number of years – it is a long-term and complex procedure. The patient needs to be organized, committed and motivated to go through the process.

9.36 How does psychoanalysis differ from psychotherapy?

Essentially, psychoanalysis is a way of understanding the mind whereas psychotherapy uses the process to resolve conflicts and provide therapy. Arising from the concept of psychoanalysis there are a range of therapeutic options available. Almost any 'talking treatment' is psychotherapy. Some therapies are superficial and brief, such as counselling, whereas others are more intensive, expensive and detailed.

Apart from the obvious differences of depth, cost and length of treatment, psychoanalysis is to do with understanding the self and resolving unconscious conflicts, thereby effecting change. Psychotherapy is much more to do with problem solving as a treatment. People undergoing analysis are not necessarily ill, and indeed the healthier they are the more they are likely to get out of analysis. You have to be pretty integrated to work hard at analysis on a regular basis for several years. Therapy implies some measure of pathology that requires treatment. Psychotherapy can be almost any form of talking treatment, ranging from one or two simple sessions of counselling up to twice-weekly therapy for a year or two. Analysis is a highly specific and structured process.

9.37 What are the different schools of psychoanalysis and does it matter which one the patient chooses?

The traditional schools are those conceived by Freud, Jung and Klein from the late 19th and early 20th century. A range of therapies have developed from these, and indeed schools of analysis are evolving all the time and new ones developing. The relationship between the client and therapist is important. The 'chemistry' between the two has to be right, as in all relationships. If there are problems between the two then the long-term relationship of therapy is unlikely to be fruitful, although some would argue that if there is a problem in the relationship then it needs to be resolved. A lot depends on which particular school of therapist is available. Many therapists are increasingly eclectic in their approach and embody the best of all therapies to suit the needs of their client. Having said that, psychoanalysis can be a very formal and often rigid process. Many patients have preconceptions about the school of analysis they wish to pursue. Embarking upon an analysis is not something that should be started without careful consideration. Kleinian therapists can be particularly threatening to a naïve patient, as they may say little or nothing during a session, making the patient do all the work. If the issue of the school of psychoanalysis becomes important, then the patient should be referred to a general psychotherapist who will be better skilled at advising on the specific school suitable to the patient's needs, as it has become a very specialized area. It is an interesting concept that the treatment that a patient gets should be determined by what is likely to benefit them, rather than what is available or what the therapist likes to practise.

9.38 Who is likely to benefit from psychoanalysis, and who should not be referred?

Those patients who want to explore their inner life in detail should be referred, and those who have thought about the matter carefully. For a psychoanalysis to work, the patient has to be organized and relatively in control of their life. They need to be able to turn up on a regular basis on time with their therapist. They need to be prepared to work hard at their problem. They need to be able to tolerate stress. They should not abuse substances nor act out by taking overdoses or get aggressive. They need to be relatively intelligent and capable of 'change'. They should not have too many distractions in their outer world. They should have a relatively stable life without too many crises. They will probably need money, as psychoanalysis is rarely available on the NHS. The people who benefit from psychoanalysis are, for example, healthcare professionals who wish to further their studies and expertise or intellectuals with an introspective bent. Disturbed chaotic individuals with severe personality disorders or drug problems are unlikely to benefit and should not be referred; although it may be quite easy to see what the problems are, that may not be enough to generate change.

Psychoanalysis is a complex therapy that explores patients' feelings about the world around them through a relationship with their therapist which reflects childhood relationships over a period of some time. It requires regular sessions, possibly once or twice or up to five times a week over a period of years. As such, it requires a degree of integration on behalf of the patient to sustain a long-term relationship, and to turn up and pay for regular sessions. Patients must be able to understand the meaning of the therapy and to tolerate some degree of stress when confronting their own painful memories and misconceptions about themselves and the world around them. Thus, not all patients are suitable to embark upon analytical therapy.

Classically, patients who do well are young, verbal, intelligent and single. They are people who still have the capacity to learn and change over a period of time, and who have the personal resources to work at their problem. Psychoanalysis works best for people with recurrent problems in their relationships with others. They can gradually change their attitudes. It is not a panacea to get to the root of all ills, and understanding the cause does not necessarily lead to the cure.

9.39 Is psychoanalysis ever available on the NHS?

Psychoanalysis is unlikely to be available, but psychoanalytic therapy may well be available especially in teaching centres. Many therapists undergoing training need to take on patients for long-term analytic therapy. This can be free or at a reasonably low cost. One of the issues around therapy is that it needs to cost the patient something, otherwise they do not appreciate it properly.

9.40 Can psychoanalysis ever be harmful?

 Yes, if patients get trapped in a relationship (and especially if the therapist then dies). They can become dependent upon their therapist. The stress may encourage them to act out. I have seen domestic relationships break down as the patient becomes increasingly involved in the therapeutic process. Psychoanalysis is not something to be embarked upon lightly.

 PATIENT QUESTIONS

9.41 What can I do to make myself feel better?

Seek help! Go and see a doctor and take advice. Contact self-help lines. Read about your depression; share your feelings with those close to you. Take exercise. Do not allow yourself to withdraw. Keep your regular routines going and take your medication regularly. Know that depression is a very treatable condition and most patients get well within a few weeks. If your depression has a particular external cause then try and deal with that. If you overwork or drink too much, take steps to control that too.

9.42 Why is psychoanalysis so expensive?

It involves frequent regular sessions over many years with a highly trained analyst. Paying for treatment is an essential part of the therapeutic mechanism, and patients have to be seen to make sacrifices in order to gain benefit (as in so many facets of life). Each session in itself is not expensive, but the costs in time and money add up.

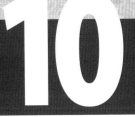

Treatment of depression – self-help and complementary therapies

10

SELF-HELP GROUPS IN DEPRESSION

10.1 What is a self-help group, and how is it organized?

Self-help groups for depression spring up like mushrooms but tend not to last very long. Often someone casts off the burden of depression, is filled with a new optimism and believes that they can then help others. As their success increases so does the strain and the burden of running such an organization, and vulnerable, depressed individuals lay all manner of pressures upon the leader of the organization, which they are not equipped to deal with.

Some groups have been set up by ex-sufferers to help other individuals learn coping skills. Support and comfort help people to deal with their problem. They are usually organized by an individual who gathers a group of fellow sufferers together. Sadly, depression is associated with a lack of sociability and social withdrawal, and this makes it less likely that depressives wish to communicate with each other.

Depression chat rooms on the Internet, on the other hand, where people can share their problems in a non-judgemental way with fellow victims, appear to be very popular.

10.2 What are the benefits of belonging to a self-help group in the treatment of depression?

Many depressed people feel very isolated and alone. They feel they are not taken seriously or validated. They lack information about treatments; they feel anxious. All of these anxieties are helped by meeting fellow victims in a non-judgemental way. The groups essentially offer support and some structure. They may even offer some therapy, although that is less common.

10.3 What are the drawbacks of self-help groups?

They often become talking shops without engineering change. They often result in great pressures on the organizers, who start off with good intentions and great enthusiasm but, as the problems of others are loaded onto their shoulders, often lack the support structures and training of professionals and soon become overwhelmed by the problems of the sufferers. Depression self-help groups particularly seem to be short lived because of the vulnerability of those that set them up. Dealing with a lot of depressed people is certainly wearing.

10.4 How can patients find out about any groups in their area?

This is difficult since groups spring up but disappear quite quickly. Information may be available in the local papers and GP surgeries. Social services may know about some. The Internet is a wonderful source of information.

Some self-help organizations such as The Depression Alliance, SANE and The Manic Depression Fellowship among others are long-standing, well-organized organizations with significant funding and substantial professional back-up. They do not usually offer support and therapy. They act mainly as information sources and political lobbying groups. (*See Appendix 6* for contact details.)

SELF-HELP

10.5 Are there any over-the-counter preparations that might help alleviate depression?

Hypericum (St John's Wort) is widely available from pharmacies and health stores. Several studies have shown that *Hypericum* is useful in the treatment of mild depression. However, it may interact with the contraceptive pill to reduce its contraceptive efficacy and can interact with other prescribed drugs. It should not be taken in pregnancy.

Some over-the-counter preparations can help insomnia. Many of these contain doses of sedating antihistamines, while others contain valerian.

COMPLEMENTARY THERAPIES

10.6 What complementary therapies are available for depression?

There are now dozens of complementary or 'alternative' therapies available. Some, like reflexology, are well-known and reasonably well-established while others are more esoteric and some are frankly bizarre in their claims. Yet others are so well-known and respected that they are considered mainstream and may even be available on the NHS. The main difficulty in assessing the claims made by practitioners of complementary therapies is that very few have been subjected to rigorous controlled trials, so it is difficult to substantiate or reject their claims of efficacy. Since most of these therapies are only available privately, it is really a case of 'buyer beware.'

10.7 What should a GP do when a patient asks for a recommendation to a complementary therapy that the GP has barely heard of?

It is important to be honest and admit that you have very little knowledge of the therapy in question. It may be appropriate to point out that there are no medical papers or controlled studies in that particular area. How has the patient heard about this particular therapy or therapist? Was it well recommended and did it seem to work appropriately? Is the patient looking for alternative treatment because he or she is dissatisfied with conventional medicine? If so, is there anything else conventional medicine can offer?

10.8 What precautions can a patient take when they consult a complementary therapist?

The best safeguard is probably personal recommendation from a friend or health professional who knows the therapist and their work. Some practitioners belong to professional bodies and can be looked up on a register. Their premises are also important. Many complementary therapists practise from smart, well-known centres with reception staff and other people working in the building. That is not to say that people who practise from their homes are not reputable – indeed many top psychoanalysts and psychotherapists do exactly that – but patients need to be aware of possible dangers and to let someone know where they are going, particularly when they are going to their first appointment. Many complementary therapists are not regulated by a professional body and don't carry professional indemnity, so getting compensation if things go wrong may be difficult.

10.9 How do we know whether any of these complementary therapies do any good – particularly in the treatment of depression?

The short answer is that we do not know anything for sure because the therapies have not been assessed with formal trials. However, there is no denying the relationship between mind, body and spirit, and many of the therapies discussed in this chapter have an uplifting effect on the spirit.

10.10 Is it the therapy itself or the therapist that effects the improvement?

It is probably both, though how much each contributes would be impossible to say. The fact that the patient has made the effort to book an appointment and is going to see someone rather than doing nothing is a positive thing. The fact that they are well-motivated enough to keep going and to keep paying is a further good sign. Then there is the time spent with the therapist. Generally, complementary consultations are longer than the 10 minutes or so available with the GP on the NHS. The therapist may take a long history and appear to be more interested or working in a more holistic way. This in itself is a powerful factor and will add towards the patient's feeling of well-being at the end of the session.

MASSAGE

10.11 What is therapeutic massage?

This is a form of massage developed by a Swedish gymnast in the late 19th century. This is why it is sometimes called Swedish massage.

10.12 How does massage work?

Touch stimulates nerve endings in the skin that send impulses to the brain – sometimes blocking chronic pain impulses in the process. Touch also stimulates the release of endorphins – the naturally occurring morphine-like substances that can alleviate pain and induce a feeling of well-being.

10.13 Is there any evidence to back up the claim that massage is beneficial?

There have been few studies – but some in the treatment of cancer patients have shown that massage can relieve anxiety, promote a feeling of well-being and relieve pain. Indeed many hospitals and palliative care units now offer massage to their patients.

10.14 Does massage have a role to play in the treatment of depression?

Massage may well have a role to play, but is not a treatment for depression in its own right. Massage undoubtedly makes the patient feel more comfortable and induces a feeling of well-being. In particular, massage may relieve the muscular tension that builds up in the neck and shoulder muscles when we are anxious and feeling stressed, and thus help to relieve that stress.

AROMATHERAPY

10.15 What is aromatherapy?

Aromatherapy is the use of special oils in therapeutic massage. These are essential oils diluted in a carrier oil and massaged into the body. Very small quantities of the essential oil are absorbed through the skin and are said to produce a therapeutic effect. In addition the oils used produce a pleasant smell during the massage.

10.16 How are the oils chosen?

The aromatherapist takes a long and detailed history and then chooses oils to relieve the specific symptoms that are worrying the patient.

10.17 Are particular oils good for depression?

Several oils are said to have antidepressant properties. These include lavender, neroli, camomile, sandalwood, eucalyptus and rose oil.

Lavender oil is said to aid sleep and have antiseptic properties as well as its antidepressant effect. Similarly, neroli oil and camomile oil also have sedative properties. As a lot of people who suffer from depression also have difficulty in sleeping, this would appear to be a beneficial effect.

10.18 Are there any pitfalls or precautions that should be taken?

As with any complementary therapy, it is important to choose a qualified experienced practitioner. The use of essential oils should be avoided in pregnancy as their safety has not been assessed. Sometimes the oil may cause an allergic reaction in the skin and should not be used. The biggest danger of seeking a complementary therapist is the risk that the patient is thereby not having effective treatment for a potentially treatable and serious condition.

LIGHT THERAPY AND SEASONAL AFFECTIVE DISORDER

10.19 What is the basis of SAD?

It is thought that natural sunlight has a therapeutic effect on the body and mind and that we suffer when we are deprived of it. In rural societies people spent a great deal of time outdoors working the land and were exposed to natural sunlight most of the day. In industrial societies we spend more time inside our homes, offices and factories where the lighting is artificial and does not contain the full spectrum of colours.

10.20 What is special about natural sunlight?

Natural sunlight contains the full spectrum of colours. In addition it contains other radiation including ultraviolet, infrared and gamma rays. This full-spectrum light is thought to influence the pineal gland, which in turn influences the production of serotonin and of melatonin during the hours of darkness. Suppression of melatonin production by treating patients with full-spectrum light is thought to be the key to treating SAD.

10.21 How can SAD be treated?

Full-spectrum lighting is thought to be effective in both treating and preventing SAD. It is important to spend as much time as possible outside in natural sunlight. Sitting outside in the garden or on the balcony or walking in the park every day can be of immense benefit. Sufferers can also sit in front of a special light box for an hour or so every day. Full-spectrum light bulbs can be bought from special suppliers for use around the home and office instead of ordinary bulbs.

10.22 Should any precautions be taken in natural sunlight?

Appropriate sunscreens should, of course, be used in fierce sunlight to prevent the burning effects of UVB radiation and the ageing effects of UVA radiation.

RELAXATION THERAPIES

10.23 Why do we need specific relaxation therapies? Do we really live in a more stressful world than our ancestors?

This is an ongoing argument – is modern-day life any more stressful than that of hunter-gatherer man? Certainly our lifestyles and expectations are very different today. We may not have to kill our own food but we often have to juggle home, family and work commitments, and it may be that we have unrealistic expectations, fuelled by the media, of a perfect happy life. While a certain amount of stress is necessary and even beneficial, excess stress can cause headaches, muscular tension, low mood, loss of libido, poor sleep and irritability.

Learning to relax and using techniques or therapies to promote relaxation helps counter the symptoms of excessive stress and leads to an improved sense of well-being and diminishing anxiety.

10.24 What types of relaxation therapy are available?

There are many aids to relaxation, from breathing techniques to listening to tapes. Many people find yoga a useful discipline in the battle against stress. Regular exercise is useful in that it stimulates the production of endorphins, which in turn have a relaxing, uplifting effect. Laughter and enjoying a good regular sexual relationship are also stress relievers. Owning a pet, usually a cat or a dog, aids relaxation and is said to relieve stress. Some people relax with music, some with dancing or drama. People may want to watch, listen or participate. Yet others enjoy a glass of wine in a warm bath or a trip to a health farm or beauty spa. It really is a case of finding what is enjoyable and relaxing and then making the time and space for it.

10.25 What is autogenic training?

This is a technique that was first developed in the early 1900s in Germany. Students are taught how to achieve a state of passive concentration rather like meditation. This can, it is said, lead to greater creativity, better communication skills and improved sporting ability, possibly because autogenic training helps to integrate left- and right-sided brain functions.

HERBALISM

10.26 Can herbalism be helpful in depression?

Many herbs are credited with helping depression. Some are the same as those used in aromatherapy. Some patients may find consulting a qualified herbalist helpful.

HOMEOPATHY

10.27 Can homeopathic treatment help depression?

As far as I know there are no specific homoeopathic remedies to treat depression. Certain remedies may, however, be helpful in relieving anxiety and promoting sleep.

 PATIENT QUESTIONS

10.28 How can depressed people help themselves?

I am glad you have asked this question, as depression is so often seen as a medical problem that should be treated or cured by medical people and methods, while the patient is passive and can do little to change the situation. The reality should be very different. Too often the depressed person stays at home, often in bed, and doesn't eat properly.

I think it is important to try to maintain a healthy lifestyle. Eating a healthy diet with lots of fruit and vegetables is essential. Going out and getting some exercise is essential. Exercise causes the release of endorphins – the naturally occurring opiates that make you feel better. Exercise also creates a sense of achievement and makes you feel better about yourself. Exercise can be free – a walk around the local park, for example. Swimming in the municipal pool or even going to the local gym may involve a small charge. Some health authorities have negotiated a prescription for exercise whereby the GP can refer the patient to the local gym without charge. Having a pet cat or dog can also lift the spirits. Dogs need to be walked, so you have a reason to go out and may meet other dog walkers in doing so. Cats do not need walking but are wonderful company and can help you relax.

Associations such as Depression Alliance and Mind can offer useful information and advice on depression and its treatment – see *Appendix 6* at the end of this book for their addresses, websites and other contact details.

10.29 Are self-help books of any use?

Some self-help books are wonderful and extremely helpful both for the sufferer and for their relatives and carers. They can explain what it feels like to be depressed and how it is not possible to 'pull up your socks' and 'snap out of it.' They can suggest self-help routines and pathways to encourage recovery. See the list of further reading at the end of this book.

10.30 What about alternative treatments? I have heard that St John's Wort is good for depression.

Alternative treatments are popular. Many people do not like to 'medicalize their problem'. They like to avoid seeing their GP if possible. Health food shops and alternative practitioners are often more sympathetic than a busy GP, and patients like to avoid the stigma of the diagnosis of depression.

Alternative treatments are usually about as good as antidepressants in mild depression. It is debatable whether antidepressants really do anything in any case for people with less severe depression. If depression is severe then you should definitely seek professional advice and take appropriate treatment. St John's Wort is probably the most extensively studied 'alternative treatment'. It appears to be as good as antidepressants in mild to moderate depression. It costs a great deal more to the patient than prescription of a modern antidepressant. I personally would prefer to take a tried and tested remedy of a pure compound than a compound of uncertain efficacy, origin and purity – but then I am biased.

10.31 What else can a depressed person do?

It is vital to avoid self-medicating with large doses of alcohol or other drugs. It is all too easy to rely on alcohol or benzodiazepine drugs such as diazepam (Valium) to help the feelings of anxiety that so frequently accompany depression or to rely on a sleeping pill to get to sleep. Sadly, all too often this leads to problems of long-term dependence as well as the original depression.

10.32 How soon will it be before I start feeling better?

This is a difficult question. Patients often feel better when they start seeking treatment and see that help is available. When they see a doctor or therapist, things can start to get sorted out and begin to improve. It may take time for depression to get better overall. Antidepressant medication tends to start working early, but the full benefit does not become apparent until three or four weeks later. Sadly, antidepressants often cause side-effects, which are maximal in the first few days and then diminish. This is before the therapeutic benefit begins, and so it is important to persist in taking medication for a few weeks if possible, abandoning it earlier only if the side-effects are really bad. Many patients stop taking antidepressants before they have had a chance to work and therefore do not get the benefit of treatment. If the antidepressant has not worked within, say, six weeks, the situation needs to be reviewed.

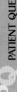

PATIENT QUESTIONS

Resistant depression

11

11.1 What is resistant depression, and how is it diagnosed?

A patient is said to be suffering from resistant depression when he or she has failed to make an adequate response to two different antidepressants given at therapeutic doses for an adequate period of time. Sadly, approximately 30% of patients fail to make an adequate response and need further treatment strategies, whether medical, social or pharmacological, to try to provide an appropriate therapeutic response.

11.2 How should treatment be altered to tackle this problem?

The first thing is a complete review of the situation to check the diagnosis, to make sure that the depression is the sort that should respond to treatment and specifically to an antidepressant, then to make sure that the patient does not have another important condition such as schizophrenia, personality disorder, substance abuse or early dementia. There may be a case for checking the bloods to exclude any covert organic cause, especially hypothyroidism. The usual therapeutic issue is then whether to increase the dose of antidepressant, possibly outside the normal recommended ranges, or to add some augmentation treatment such as lithium, tryptophan or thyroxine or possibly an additional antidepressant. There may be a case for considering psychotherapy if psychological factors are to the fore, or if the depression is severe then ECT might be considered either on an outpatient or an inpatient basis. Options for the treatment of resistant depression are listed in *Box 8.1*.

Resistant depression is a serious condition that warrants vigorous treatment. The earlier the treatment is instituted the better the prognosis. If left untreated for too long, patients can become chronic. It is really the treatment province of a specialist, and patients should be referred on early rather than waiting until it is too late.

11.3 What proportion of patients treated with an antidepressant fail to show an adequate response?

About 30% of patients fail to make an adequate response depending upon definition and how this is measured. On the one hand, antidepressants are quite effective, but on the other they are not much better than placebo and not everyone benefits, allowing a substantial proportion of patients to remain substantially impaired. With vigorous treatment possibly another 10–15% will improve. There still remain 10–15% of patients who do not make an adequate response. With these, one has to await either natural resolution of the condition or accept that depression is indeed a condition of high morbidity and that there is an unfortunate minority who have a poor prognosis and will remain chronically unwell.

11.4 How big a problem is non-compliance with medication?

Compliance, or 'concordance with a therapeutic programme' as it is now known, is a major problem. About a third of patients do not cash the prescription they are offered. They see medication as inappropriate treatment for their depression. Those patients who get their prescriptions very often do not take the medication on a regular basis as necessary. A further proportion of patients fail to take the full therapeutic course and stop before the medication has time to act. Another group of patients stop the medication as soon as they begin to feel better but then lapse into a state of semi-improvement in which their condition is just bearable. Many patients develop minor side-effects in the first few days of medication and stop the treatment, especially if it has not been explained to them that side-effects occur in the first few days before the therapeutic response but tend to wane after a few days. There is a general reluctance among patients to take medication, which of course reduces the impact and benefits of antidepressant medication substantially.

11.5 What can be done to minimize non-compliance?

A good doctor–patient relationship and time spent with the patient to understand their needs and expectations are crucial. Time to explain what medication and other therapeutic avenues can realistically offer helps. If we are talking about antidepressants, then the benefits of medication need to be explained. Information sheets will help. Patients need to be reassured that antidepressants are not 'addictive' despite what they have read in the popular press. They need to be told about early side-effects that may emerge before the therapeutic benefit is established. The patient needs to be reviewed in a positive manner and further encouraged to persist with treatment if they have not made a good response within a few weeks. Compliance is probably better with the more modern medications where side-effects are less. Simple dosage requirements where only one tablet a day needs to be taken help. Patients have become increasingly sensitized to side-effects these days and have become preoccupied with even minor side-effects which they would put up with if they really believed that the treatment would work. Patients appear to be more concerned about possible side-effects than therapeutic benefits. The benefits of treatment are generally high, and the patient should be encouraged to persist.

11.6 How do you link into already very established depressed patients?

Sadly depression is a chronic condition in a substantial minority of patients (maybe 15%). These patients have to some degree a 'resistant depression' or dysthymia. They are in need of full evaluation and appropriate treatment in order not only to potentially cure them but also to alleviate at least part of their symptoms and prevent a deterioration of their condition. The first thing to establish is that they have been correctly diagnosed as having a depressive illness rather than some other cause of depression either resulting from lifestyle, drug abuse, a poor domestic situation, physical illness, or some other unrecognized mental illness such as anxiety.

The second issue is to make sure they have had optimal treatment with full doses of antidepressants and also an opportunity to have psychological treatment, according to CBT principles, rather than simple counselling. It is important that the patients have complied with and adhered to their treatment – not only that it has been prescribed but that they have taken their medication properly and they have worked on their therapy.

If patients remain depressed despite full attempts at treatment, they should be referred to a specialist with an interest in resistant depression. There are many interesting pharmacological and therapeutic techniques available to deal with this problem. On a pharmacological line there are augmentation treatments with thyroxine, lithium and other combinations of antidepressants. Patients should not stay on the same antidepressant indefinitely if it is not helping them; they should be switched or have their doses changed, and this needs to be done in a structured way. If the primary-care practitioner is not confident in dealing with these issues the patient should be referred to a specialist. Probably half of patients with resistant depression should improve at least to some degree with appropriate treatment. Beyond that, if all fails, then support, comfort and reassurance should remain the backstop treatment until, one hopes, matters resolve themselves.

Suicide and self-harm

12

12.1 How common is suicide in the UK?

The reduction of suicide rates has been one of the key targets in the British Government's 'Health of the Nation Statement 1992'. The scale of the problem is immense. In the UK there are just over 6500 suicides annually, and this is almost double the death toll from road traffic accidents; 160 000 attempt suicide each year, although not all of these actually try to kill themselves.

12.2 Which patients are most at risk of suicide?

This is a very worrying area for GPs and one for which we sometimes feel poorly prepared. Preventing suicide is obviously the main aim, but this may be difficult to do in practice. How do you spot the patient who is truly suicidal in the middle of a busy surgery? Are the patients who talk about it the most the ones who are most likely to attempt to kill themselves? Is suicide the only way out for patients with long-standing misery and depression? These are all difficult questions.

Three-quarters of successful suicides are by men, although women outnumber men when it comes to episodes of 'self-harm' or 'suicide attempts'. Other risk factors include previous attempts and statement of intent, although some people talk repeatedly about suicide without any intention of completing the act. Old, lonely men who suffer from painful illnesses are particularly at risk, as are those with depressive disorders, especially when there are severe mood changes with insomnia and anorexia with weight loss. Patients are at particular risk during the phase of recovery when energy levels return and they can act on their bad thoughts. Hopelessness is a predictor of suicide.

Other risk factors include alcohol dependence, especially where social damage and drug dependence is associated with it, epilepsy and abnormal personalities. Suicide is particularly likely in young schizophrenic men with severe illnesses and intellectual deterioration.

Being in the medical or farming professions carries an increased suicide risk causing great concern, and veterinarians come top of the list of suicide risk. Alcohol is important as a contributor to suicide.

Risk factors for suicide are listed in *Box 12.1*. An ascending hierarchy of indicators of suicide risk is given in *Box 12.2*.

BOX 12.1 Risk factors for suicide

Male

Older age group

Disturbed family background

- Psychiatric history in family (especially interaction with psychotic parent)
- History of suicide in family
- Death of a parent
- Parental divorce, separation, continual conflict between parents
- Negative parental messages to child (e.g. child is a burden or is failing to live up to expectations)
- Efforts of child to express unhappiness, failure or frustration are unacceptable to parents
- Sexual, physical or emotional abuse
- Child forced into 'parental' role
- Parents fail to meet child's emotional needs

Physical illness

Psychiatric illness

Alcohol/drug abuse (history in approximately 50% of suicides)

Difficulties with schooling

Sexual-identity problems

Problems with individuating from family

Destructive peer pressure

Birthdays (suicide risk increases three-fold during 2 weeks after a birthday)

Average/high intelligence (NB: Suicides in tertiary education are relatively common, possible due to pressures related to the academic environment)

Dispute with/rejection by boyfriend or girlfriend

Variety of disturbed responses and behaviours (depressive mood and ideas, preoccupation with death, deliberate self-harm, social withdrawal, risk taking or antisocial behaviour, multiple somatic complaints, eating disorders)

12.3 What are the most common methods of suicide in this country?

People tend to use what is available to them. Medications from the medicines cabinet or analgesics are widely used. Other methods of suicide involve hanging – a common method in institutions – self-poisoning with psychotropic drugs among outpatients, and using motorcar exhausts or jumping are also effective means. Farmers are particularly at risk of using shotguns because they have access to them.

BOX 12.2 An ascending hierarchy of indicators of suicide risk

- Does the patient feel life is not worth living?
- Does he or she wish to go to sleep and never wake up?
- Does he or she wish to die suddenly or be killed in an accident?
- Is there a preoccupation with death and dying?
- Are there vague thoughts of suicide?
- Do the patient's thoughts centre on methods of suicide?
- Has the patient plans to commit suicide?

12.4 What is the difference between suicide and attempted suicide? Is it simply that the first is successful and the second is not? Is it a measure of efficacy or is it more a measure of intent?

Parasuicide is suicidal-like behaviour, otherwise known as 'deliberate self-harm' (DSH). When dealing with these patients it soon becomes clear that, although they take an overdose or otherwise risk their lives, the real intention is not to kill themselves. Theirs is more of an impulsive act, a cry for help or an attempt at manipulating a situation. The intention to kill themselves is not very strong and therefore failed suicides are called parasuicides. They are often fuelled by alcohol. Relationship problems are often a factor.

Parasuicide is about 15 times more common in men and 30 times more common in women than successful suicide. About 1–2% of parasuicides kill themselves within a 2-year period – a death rate some 50–100 times higher than that of the general population. The eventual death rate of people who indulge in parasuicide may be as high as 20%, so it is not without risk as well as being a clumsy way of dealing with emotional difficulties.

12.5 What aspects of a patient's history or behaviour should alert me to the possibility of suicide or self-harm?

A history of suicide attempts, depression, drug abuse, unemployment, mental illness and social isolation. Most depressed patients will admit to some suicidal ideation, but it is the level of ideation that is important. For example, if the patient has made plans and already acted on them, such as working out what the lethal dose of medication is and taking steps to obtain it, and is now just waiting for one event, such as his wife going away, to complete the act, this is a very high suicide risk. Simply wondering whether life is really worth living at a philosophical level can be regarded as a low risk. Patients generally welcome being asked about suicidal intention, and doctors should not be frightened of asking about it. It does not put the idea into the patient's head. Patients often feel relieved to discuss their worst fears. *Box 12.3* outlines how to interview a suicidal patient.

> **BOX 12.3 How to interview a suicidal patient**
> ■ Interview in a quiet uninterrupted setting
> ■ Do not hurry
> ■ Initiate interview with non-directive open questioning, allowing ventilation of issues and feelings important to the patient
> ■ Use language that is appropriate for patient, take account of variation in cultural values and religious beliefs
> ■ Build up trust and rapport quickly
> ■ Avoid brusque, challenging judgemental approach (observe where possible the Rogerian principles of warmth, empathic understanding and unconditional positive regard)
> ■ Listen to what the patient says
> ■ Allow repetitive discussion of issues if necessary
> ■ Take note of non-verbal behaviour that may be of significance regarding suicide risk
> ■ Evaluate recent events
> ■ Take a full psychiatric, medical and social history
> ■ Evaluate the mental state
> ■ Beware of hazards in assessment
> ■ Carefully evaluate suicidal motivation
> ■ Consider use of risk questionnaire

From a statistical point of view, people at particular risk are elderly, depressed males who have alcohol problems and are socially isolated. They feel hopeless and often have physical illness. Having a medical background is also a risk factor. In simple terms, an elderly, widowed, depressed doctor with a terminal illness and socially isolated, has the means of killing him- or herself and is at considerable risk. Another group at high risk for suicide includes young psychotic patients who appear to be recovering and in whom insight is returning. For both groups the greatest risk of suicide is at a time when they make a partial recovery. Their energy level increases but their sense of despair remains, and this combination of events makes them particularly vulnerable.

Most people who kill themselves have contact with a doctor in the preceding weeks. People who ultimately kill themselves are often under-treated for their depression, having been given inadequate courses of antidepressants or none at all.

12.6 What can be done to prevent suicide?

This question has been addressed by the *National Suicide Prevention Strategy for England*, published by the Department of Health. The document deals with reducing the availability and lethality of suicide methods, such as better monitoring of disturbed inmates in prison and reducing the ability to hang oneself from a suitable hook while in hospital being treated for depression. One of the best ways of preventing suicide is to make the means more difficult to access, often by placing physical barriers in the way or removing potential weapons, or limiting the amount of pills that patients can obtain easily. Prescribing antidepressants that have low toxicity in overdose is an obvious safety strategy.

Treating depression vigorously should have an impact, as should close monitoring of people who are noted to be suicidal risks. When all is said and done, prevention of suicide is a difficult task for which there is no easy prescription.

12.7 Are there any protective factors where suicide is concerned?

Protective factors include: a secure and safe environment, learning skills in problem solving and impulse control; learning how to deal with conflict resolution; family and community support; avoiding alcohol; and easy access to adequate mental healthcare. Cultural and religious beliefs that discourage suicide may also be protective.

12.8 How common is suicide in the elderly, and what can be done to prevent it?

Suicide statistics in general are difficult to interpret because suicide is generally under-reported as a result of its legal definition and the social stigma attached. Thus they represent a gross underestimate of the true picture. The official figures for England and Wales are 121 suicides per million males, and 57 per million females. Suicide rates increase significantly in the elderly, where attempts at self-harm are much more likely to be aimed at suicide than as a suicidal gesture. Eight percent of men and 3% of women who have made a suicide attempt when aged over 55 have been shown ultimately to kill themselves.

The vast majority of elderly suicide attempters are clinically depressed, so the most important preventive measure is to diagnose and treat their depression effectively. Most people who kill themselves have been seen by a doctor in the weeks prior to their death. Thus, prompt medical, social and psychological treatment for their depressive states is important. Doctors should especially be wary of patients with significant self-neglect and those who abuse alcohol.

12.9 How should I react if I think a patient is really suicidal?

The patient should be admitted to hospital immediately or at least managed in a safe environment. Unfortunately, except in extreme cases, suicidal patients rarely give real indications that they are about to harm themselves.

People who take overdoses or make parasuicide attempts usually do it for some ulterior motive rather than actually to kill themselves. If there is a risk of suicide or a suicide attempt, then prescriptions should be limited to one week's supply at a time of a safe antidepressant and the patient monitored carefully until there has been an adequate improvement in his or her clinical state. The people who kill themselves tend to be either elderly isolated males, or young psychotic patients who have the insight to realize that their future lives are grim and decide they no longer wish to carry on living. Family support is helpful in monitoring the situation. Unfortunately, it is often the silent, non-complaining person who commits suicide rather than the dramatic hysteric who projects all his anxieties onto the doctor and then feels better himself or herself as the crisis develops.

Refer to the mental-health team for urgent assessment if in doubt.

PATIENT QUESTION

12.10 What should I do if I think someone I know is suicidal?

Don't keep your fears to yourself and feel guilty about it. Speak to the person you are concerned about. Speak to the principal carer involved, or to the healthcare professional involved – someone who is able to evaluate and act on the information. Suicidal thoughts are common and rarely acted apon but must be taken seriously and evaluated via a risk assessment. The patient needs to know that their despair is acknowledged, that they are safe and supported and that they will be getting help not only for their depression but for any problems that they think cause their depression. Don't carry the secret yourself.

The Mental Health Act

13.1 What is the Mental Health Act?

The Mental Health Act is a series of laws relating to the compulsory treatment of patients in hospital. It is essentially there to deal with how patients can receive the benefits of treatment when their mental illness or condition prevents them from obtaining it themselves. The most recent legislation is the 1983 Act but legislation has built up over the last hundred years or so from the lunacy laws. The laws have changed in response to prevailing social climate and attitudes to mental illness. The previous legislation, the 1959 Act, was about affording mentally ill patients the same rights, privileges and access to treatments as physically ill patients. The 1983 Act focused more on the rights of patients, and the latest revision appears to reflect public concerns over safety and the dangers of mentally ill patients in the community. The pendulum is again swinging in favour of public protection. With all such legislation, the rights of the patients to self-determination and their human rights of expression have to be balanced against the rights to the benefits of treatment and to the protection of themselves and society.

13.2 What proportion of people are detained in hospital under the Mental Health Act?

Less than 5% of mentally ill patients are detained in hospital under the Mental Health Act. Those patients who are detained tend to suffer from psychotic illnesses – mostly schizophrenia. Very few patients with depressive illnesses are detained in hospital. On the other hand, with the current closure of beds and policies of only admitting the most severely ill patients to hospital, approximately 50% of patients in acute psychiatric beds at any one time are detained under the Mental Health Act.

13.3 What is the purpose of the Act, and whom is it designed to protect?

The Act is designed to enable patients to have treatment, and a secondary issue is to protect patients and the public. The balance between these two issues shifts from time to time. The 1959 legislation had the focus of affording patients free access to treatment even if mental illness prevented them accessing care. The current Act is designed to protect the individual who may be unable to get help. The care programme approach is designed to provide care more formally for those who are severely ill where the services appear to be disorganized. There are now duties of aftercare imposed on health and social services for patients who have been detained. It is also designed to protect individuals and the public who may be threatened by mentally ill individuals. It is also there to protect patients from exploitation and coercion by healthcare professionals.

13.4 What parts of the Act am I most likely to need?

There are four main sections that deal with admission of patients to hospital (*see Table 13.1*).

IF I WANTED TO ADMIT A VERY DEPRESSED PATIENT WHOM I THOUGHT WAS LIKELY TO KILL HIM/HERSELF BUT WHO REFUSED TO GO IN VOLUNTARILY?

The most appropriate section for a depressed patient who is suicidal is Section 2. This is a 28-day order for 'assessment and treatment'. It requires an application by a social worker on behalf of the nearest relative, and two medical recommendations: ideally one by the GP who should know the patient previously and the second by a hospital specialist with expertise in psychiatry 'approved under Section 12'.

TABLE 13.1 Sections of the Mental Health Act

Section	Duration of detention	Signatories	Comment
Section 4	Up to 72 hours	Social worker and any medical practitioner	An emergency section when time does not allow more formal assessment
Section 2	Up to 28 days	Social worker, GP and psychiatrist	The standard treatment and assessment section
Section 3	Up to 6 months	Social worker acting on behalf of nearest relative, GP and specialist	Treatment order for patients with established illness. Duty of aftercare
Section 136	Up to 72 hours	Police officer	To enable patient to be taken from a public place to a place of safety to be examined by a doctor and social worker
Section 37	Up to 6 months renewable	Judge or magistrate	Upon the advice of a medical practitioner and a specialist An order imposed by a court upon a mentally abnormal offender

IF I WANTED TO ADMIT A PATIENT WITH A SERIOUS PSYCHOTIC ILLNESS WHO HAS BEEN REFUSING TO TAKE HIS/HER MEDICATION AND WHOSE CONDITION WAS GIVING SERIOUS CAUSE FOR CONCERN TO RELATIVES AND NEIGHBOURS?

For a psychotic patient with a long-standing illness which has already been assessed and who is known to the services, a Section 3 treatment order, lasting up to 6 months, with a duty of aftercare would be the appropriate order since the patient is already diagnosed and has long-term needs after leaving hospital.

13.5 Whose duty is it to enforce the Mental Health Act once the relevant papers are signed?

It is the duty of the social worker to convey the patient to hospital, but the assistance of the police may be called on if needed.

13.6 What right of appeal do patients have if they feel they have been detained against their best interests?

On admission to hospital patients are served with a form outlining their rights of appeal. They should also have their rights explained to them. There should be public notices available on the ward on how to access a lawyer. The patients should be helped in any appeal they wish to make. The appeal should occur within a couple of weeks under Section 2 and within a few weeks under Section 3, and should be heard by a Mental Health Act tribunal. There may be instances when patients can also appeal to the hospital managers.

Patients who appeal will be examined by an independent psychiatrist on behalf of the tribunal, and they may also have legal representation.

If patients have treatment enforced upon them beyond 3 months they have to either agree to the treatment or the psychiatrist has to seek an independent opinion from a Mental Health Act commissioner (an independent psychiatrist) as to whether the treatment is appropriate and, if so, the treatment has to be 'authorized'.

13.7 What are the proposed changes to the Mental Health Act?

The legislation is currently before parliament and is undergoing consultation. The main proposed changes reflect the climate of increased concerns over protection to the public. One of the two main proposed changes concerns people with personality disorders for whom there is no obvious treatment. They could be detained in hospital prior to having committed any offence. The concern over this is that there are limited resources available at best in the psychiatric services, and the view is that these should be targeted where they can be most effective. The infringement of human rights by preventive detention for those who have not committed any crimes and for whom there is no specific treatment is another issue. The benefit to the public would be the protection of the public against individuals who are highly likely to be dangerous. Potential serious sex offenders might come under this category, as would psychopaths and possibly drug addicts and alcoholics.

The other proposed change would be a 'community treatment order'. Currently patients can (with certain exceptions) only be treated inside a hospital, but once they have left hospital, although there is a duty of the psychiatric services to provide care, there is not a duty for the patients to accept that treatment (usually depot antipsychotic medication to prevent relapses).

The new proposals would require a patient under some circumstances to accept treatment in the community to prevent them becoming sick rather than waiting for them to become sick again and then being admitted to hospital. The main concern over this is the practical problem of forcing patients to accept treatment in their own homes, which may be difficult and distasteful.

There are other, more complex issues to be addressed, including the severity of a condition that would justify sectioning, and the level of non-medical involvement in making decisions about whom to admit and whom to discharge.

13.8 What is a community treatment order, and how does it work?

A community treatment order would require patients to receive and accept treatment in the community while mentally well in order to prevent a deterioration in their condition requiring admission to hospital or causing concerns and a danger to themselves or others. This is controversial insofar as it requires coercion of people who are essentially healthy but are at risk of relapsing into an illness. The alternative view is that it prevents people from becoming ill when, through lack of insight, they are not aware of that risk. This primarily relates to schizophrenic patients on long-term antipsychotic medication. There are major objections to such an order on the grounds of civil liberties and also by nurses and other healthcare professionals who have to administer the treatment and who do not see themselves as gaolers and agents of social control, but as providers of healthcare. On the other hand the benefits of community care can only be truly effective if the patient is mentally stable while being rehabilitated in the community. Coercion has been argued to be a cheap alternative to a comprehensive community support service, to work alongside the patient.

Although not generally discussed, there are several community treatment orders in place. Seriously mentally ill offenders, for example schizophrenic murderers, can after a period of stabilization in hospital be discharged on licence under Section 37/41 of the Mental Health Act which requires them to have regular supervision and medication in the community, and if they refuse treatment they are liable to be recalled to hospital. Through this procedure, many potentially very dangerous individuals can live safely and with substantial liberty in the community. Alternatively, there are probation orders with a condition of treatment attached to them, and if patients do not accept treatment, they are liable to go before the courts and be imprisoned. A third form of treatment order is a guardianship order where social services can apply for a patient to reside at a certain place or attend a certain clinic, but they cannot require the patient to accept treatment while there, and so guardianship orders are rarely invoked.

 PATIENT QUESTION

13.9   If I am admitted to hospital will they keep me there against my wishes?

Almost certainly no. Very few depressed patients are kept in hospital under the Mental Health Act against their wishes. To be detained involuntarily, you have to be seriously mentally ill and to be a significant risk to yourself (possibly suicidal) or others and to refuse treatment. Detention would need the consent of your nearest relative. There are well-established routes of appeal against detention. It is rare for depressed patients to be kept in hospital against their wishes. The main preoccupation of doctors and nurses is how to discharge the patient at the earliest opportunity rather than filling up scarce hospital beds.

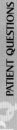

APPENDIX 1
Hamilton Depression Rating Scale

Hamilton depression rating scale		
Patient name	**Date**	
	Score range	**Score**
Depressed mood	0–4	
Guilt	0–4	
Suicide	0–4	
Insomnia – early	0–2	
Insomnia – middle	0–2	
Insomnia – late	0–2	
Work and activities	0–4	
Retardation	0–4	
Agitation	0–4	
Anxiety psychic	0–4	
Anxiety somatic	0–4	
Somatic symptoms: gastrointestinal	0–2	
Somatic symptoms: general	0–2	
Genital symptoms	0–2	
Hypochondriasis	0–4	
Loss of weight	0–2	
Insight	0–2	
Total score		

▲

Fig. A1.1 Hamilton Depression Rating Scale score chart. Reproduced from Hamilton, M. Journal of Neurology, Neurosurgery and Psychiatry, 1960; 23:56–62, with permission from the BMJ Publishing Group.

APPENDIX 2
Geriatric Depression Rating Scale

Geriatric Depression Rating Scale (GDS) - Short form

instructions

Undertake the test orally. Obtain a clear yes or no answer. If necessary, repeat the question

	Question	Yes	No
1	Are you basically satisfied with your life?		
2	Have you dropped many of your activities and interests?		
3	Do you feel your life is empty?		
4	Do you often get bored?		
5	Are you in good spirits most of the time?		
6	Are you afraid that something bad is going to happen to you?		
7	Do you feel happy most of the time?		
8	Do you often feel helpless?		
9	Do you prefer to stay at home, rather than going out and doing new things?		
10	Do you feel you have more problems with memory than most?		
11	Do you think it is wonderful to be alive now?		
12	Do you feel pretty worthless the way you are now?		
13	Do you feel full of energy?		
14	Do you feel that your situation is hopeless?		
15	Do you think that most people are better off than you are?		

A score for each item as listed scores one

A score in excess of 4 is probably depressed

A score in excess of 9 is almost certainly depressed

Fig. A2.1 The Geriatric Depression Rating Scale (GDS).

APPENDIX 3
Hospital Anxiety and Depression Scale

Doctors are aware that emotions play an important part in most illnesses. If your doctor knows about these feelings, he/she will be able to help you more.
This questionnaire is designed to help your doctor to know how you feel. Read each item and circle the score beside the reply which comes closest to how you have been feeling in the past week.
Don't take too long over your replies; your immediate reaction to each item will probably be more accurate than a long thought out response.

Circle one score per item

D / A	I feel tense or 'wound up':	D / A	I feel as if I am slowed down:
3	Most of the time	3	Nearly all the time
2	A lot of the time	2	Very often
1	From time to time, occasionally	1	Sometimes
0	Not at all	0	Not at all

D / A	I still enjoy the things I used to enjoy:	D / A	I get a sort of frightened feeling like 'butterflies' in the stomach:
0	Definitely as much		
1	Not quite so much	0	Not at all
2	Only a little	1	Occasionally
3	Hardly at all	2	Quite often
		3	Very often

	I get a sort of frightened feeling as if something awful is about to happen:		I have lost interest in my appearance:
3	Very definitely and quite badly	3	Definitely
2	Not quite so much now	2	I don't take so much care as I should
1	Definitely not so much now	1	I may not take quite as much care
0	Not at all	0	I take just as much care as ever

	I can laugh and see the funny side of things:		I feel restless as if I have to be on the move:
0	As much as I always could	3	Very much indeed
1	Not quite so much now	2	Quite a lot
2	Definitely not so much now	1	Not very much
3	Not at all	0	Not at all

	Worrying thoughts go through my mind:		I look forward with enjoyment to things:
		0	As much as I ever did
3	A great deal of the time	1	Rather less than I used to
2	A lot of the time	2	Definitely less than I used to
1	From time to time but not too often	3	Hardly at all
0	Only occasionally		

	I feel cheerful:		I get sudden feelings of panic:
		3	Very often indeed
3	Not at all	2	Quite often
2	Not often	1	Not very often
1	Sometimes	0	Not at all
0	Most of the time		

	I can sit at ease and feel relaxed:		I can enjoy a good book or radio or TV programme:
0	Definitely	0	Often
1	Usually	1	Sometimes
2	Not often	2	Not often
3	Not at all	3	Very seldom

Now check to be sure you have answered all the questions

Total score and grading

Total score: Anxiety _____ Depression _____
Grading: 0–7 Non-case   8–10 Borderline case   11+ Case

Fig. A3.1 Hospital Anxiety and Depression Scale (HADS), which is completed by the patient. The scoring system has been added to the questionnaire. (From Zigmond A S, Snaith R P 1983 The hospital anxiety and depression scale. Acta Psychiatrica Scandinavica 67:361–370.)

As you have recently had a baby, we would like to know how you are feeling.
Please **underline the statement** that comes closest to how you have felt IN THE PAST 7 DAYS, not just how you feel today. Here is an example, already completed.

1. I have felt happy:
Yes, all the time
Yes, most of the time
No, not very often
No, not at all

This would mean: 'I have felt happy most of the time' during the past week.
Please complete the other questions in the same way:

In the past 7 days

1. I have been able to laugh and see the funny side of things:
As much as I always could
Not quite so much now
Definitely not so much now
Not at all

2. I have looked forward with enjoyment to things
As much as I ever did
Rather less than I used to
Definitely less than I used to
Hardly at all

*3. I have blamed myself unnecessarily when things went wrong:
Yes, most of the time
Yes, some of the time
Not very often
No, never

4. I have been anxious or worried for no good reason:
No, not at all
Hardly ever
Yes, sometimes
Yes, very often

*5. I have felt scared or panicky for no very good reason:
Yes, quite a lot
Yes, sometimes
No, not much
No, not at all

*6. Things have been getting on top of me:
Yes, most of the time I haven't been able to cope at all
Yes, sometimes I haven't been coping as well as usual
No, most of the time I have coped quite well
No, I have been coping as well as ever

*7. I have been so unhappy that I have had difficulty sleeping:
Yes, most of the time
Yes, sometimes
Not very often
No, not at all

*8. I have felt sad or miserable:
Yes, most of the time
Yes, quite often
Not very often
No, not at all

*9. I have been so unhappy that I have been crying:
Yes, most of the time
Yes, quite often
Only occasionally
No, never

*10. The thought of harming myself has occurred to me:
Yes, quite often
Sometimes
Hardly ever
Never

Instructions for users

The mother is asked to underline the response that comes closest to how she has been feeling in the previous 7 days.

All ten items must be completed.

Care should be taken to avoid the possibility of the mother discussing her answers with others.

The mother should complete the scale herself, unless she has limited English or has difficulty with reading.

The EPDS may be used at 6–8 weeks to screen postnatal women. The child health clinic, postnatal check-up or a home visit may provide suitable opportunities for completion.

Response categories are scored 0, 1, 2 and 3 according to increased severity of the symptoms, items marked with an asterisk are reverse scored (3, 2, 1 and 0). The total score is calculated by adding together the scores for each of the ten items.

Mothers who score above a threshold of 12/13 should be further assessed.

For routine use in primary care, it might be appropriate to assess further those mothers scoring above a threshold of 9/10.

The score should not override clinical judgement, and a careful clinical assessment should be carried out to confirm the diagnosis.

The scale indicates how the mother has felt during the previous week, and in doubtful cases it may be usefully repeated after 2 weeks.

The scale will not detect mothers with anxiety neuroses, phobias or personality disorders.

▲

Fig. A4.1 Edinburgh Postnatal Depression Scale. (From Cox J, Holden J, Sagovsky R 1987 Detection of postnatal depression. Development of the 10-item Edinburgh Postnatal Depression Scale. British Journal of Psychiatry 150:782–786, with permission from the Royal College of Psychiatrists.)

APPENDIX 5
Switching or stopping antidepressants

The following table gives, for a variety of antidepressants, details of precautions to be taken when stopping or switching a tricyclic to a selective serotonin reuptake inhibitor, and vice-versa.

TABLE A5.1 Antidepressants – swapping and stopping

To / From	MAOIs / hydrazines	Tranyl-cypromine	Tricyclics	Citalopram	Fluoxetine	Paroxetine	Sertraline	Trazodone	Moclobemide	Reboxetine	Venlafaxine	Mirtazapine
Sertraline	Withdraw and wait for 2 weeks[a]	Withdraw and wait for 2 weeks	Cross taper cautiously with very low dose of tricyclic[b]	Withdraw then start citalopram	Withdraw then start fluoxetine	Withdraw then start paroxetine	–	Withdraw before starting trazodone/ nefazodone	Withdraw and wait at least 2 weeks	Cross taper cautiously	Withdraw then start venlafaxine at 37.5 mg/day	Withdraw before starting mirtazapine cautiously
Trazodone	Withdraw and wait at least 1 week	Withdraw and wait at least 1 week	Cross taper cautiously with very low dose of tricyclic	Withdraw then start citalopram	Withdraw then start fluoxetine	Withdraw then start paroxetine	Withdraw then start sertraline	–	Withdraw and wait at least 1 week	Withdraw then start reboxetine at 2 mg b.d. and increase cautiously	Withdraw then start venlafaxine at 37.5 mg/day	Withdraw before starting mirtazapine cautiously
Moclobemide	Withdraw and wait 24 hours	Withdraw and wait 24 hours	Withdraw and wait 24 hours	Withdraw and wait 24 hours	Withdraw and wait 24 hours	Withdraw and wait 24 hours	Withdraw and wait 24 hours	Withdraw and wait 24 hours	–	Withdraw and wait 24 hours	Withdraw and wait 24 hours	Withdraw and wait 24 hours
Reboxetine	Withdraw and wait at least 1 week	Withdraw and wait at least 1 week	Cross taper cautiously	Cross taper cautiously	Cross taper cautiously	Cross taper cautiously	Cross taper cautiously	Cross taper cautiously	Withdraw and wait at least 1 week	–	Cross taper cautiously	Cross taper cautiously
Venlafaxine	Withdraw and wait at least 1 week	Withdraw and wait at least 1 week	Cross taper cautiously with very low dose of tricyclic[b]	Cross taper cautiously Start with 10 mg/day	Cross taper cautiously Start with 20 mg every other day	Cross taper cautiously Start with 10 mg/day	Cross taper cautiously Start with 25 mg/day	Cross taper cautiously	Withdraw and wait at least 1 week	Cross taper cautiously	–	Withdraw before starting mirtazapine cautiously

TABLE A5.1 Antidepressants – swapping and stopping—contd

From \ To	MAOIs/hydrazines	Tranyl-cypromine	Tricyclics	Citalopram	Fluoxetine	Paroxetine	Sertraline	Trazodone	Moclobemide	Reboxetine	Venlafaxine	Mirtazapine
Mirtazapine	Withdraw and wait for 1 week	Withdraw and wait for 1 week	Withdraw then start tricyclic	Withdraw then start citalopram	Withdraw then start fluoxetine	Withdraw then start paroxetine	Withdraw then start sertraline	Withdraw then start trazodone / nefazodone	Withdraw and wait 1 week	Withdraw then start reboxetine	Withdraw then start venlafaxine	–
Stopping[d]	Reduce over 4 weeks	Reduce over 4 weeks	Reduce over 4 weeks	Reduce over 4 weeks	At 20 mg/day, just stop[c] At 40 mg/day reduce over 2 weeks	Reduce over 4 weeks or longer, if necessary[e]	Reduce over 4 weeks	Reduce over 4 weeks	Reduce over 4 weeks	Reduce over 4 weeks	Reduce over 4 weeks, or longer if necessary[e]	Reduce over 4 weeks

[a] Abrupt switching is possible but not recommended.
[b] Do not co-administer clomipramine and SSRIs or venlafaxine. Withdraw clomipramine before starting.
[c] Beware interactions with fluoxetine may still occur for 5 weeks after stopping fluoxetine, because of long half-life.
[d] See general guidelines.
[e] Withdrawal effects seem to be more pronounced. Slow withdrawal over 1–3 months may be necessary.
From Taylor D et al (eds) 2001 The Maudsley prescribing guidelines, 6th edn. Martin Dunitz, London, with permission from Taylor and Francis.

APPENDIX 6
Useful websites and other sources of further information

Professional organizations

PriMHE

The Old Stables

2a Laurel Avenue

Twickenham

Middlesex

TW1 4JA

http://www.primhe.org

Aims to provide mental health support, services, resources, education and training to help primary-care professionals and staff achieve and deliver the best standards of mental healthcare. Lists links to useful articles, recommended training resources, and sells a resource pack for primary care practitioners.

The Royal College of Psychiatrists

National Headquarters

17 Belgrave Square

London

SW1X 8PG

Email: rcpsych@rcpsych.ac.uk

Tel: 020 7235 2351

Fax: 020 7245 1231

http://www.rcpsych.ac.uk/info/help/anxiety/

Gives brief overview of condition and points to the sources of further help (some of which are included in this list). Provides information leaflets and a learning audiotape pack for the general public.

The Royal Australian and New Zealand College of Psychiatrists

309 La Trobe Street

Melbourne

Victoria 3000

Australia

Tel: +613 9640 0646

Fax: +613 9642 5652

Email: ranzcp@ranzcp.org

http://www.ranzcp.org/

The Resources section provides access to medical databases, documents, external links and other resources relevant to psychiatry and mental health. A range of information on psychiatric illness and mental healthcare suitable for allied professionals and the general public is also provided within this section.

National Institute of Mental Health (NIMH)
http://www.nimh.nih.gov/

US government site. Includes descriptions of anxiety, panic, and related disorders and their treatment for non-medical readers, as well as access to clinical trials and research information for the practitioner.

National Mental Health Association (NMHA)
http://www.nmha.org/

Non-profit organization addressing all aspects of mental health and mental illness in the USA

American Psychiatric Association
http://www.psych.org/

Community Psychiatric Nurses Association
http://www.cpna.org.uk/index1.html

Mentality
http://www.mentality.org.uk/

UK charity dedicated solely to the promotion of mental health. Aims to work in partnership with organizations to form and implement mental health promotion policy at local, regional or national level.

Mental-health charities and patient organizations

Mental Health Foundation

UK Office:
7th Floor, 83 Victoria Street
London
SW1H 0HW
Tel: + 44 (0) 20 7802 0300
Fax: + 44 (0) 20 7802 0301
Email: mhf@mhf.org.uk
http://www.mentalhealth.org.uk

Scotland Office:
5th Floor
Merchants House
30 George Square
Glasgow
G2 1EG
Tel: + 44 (0) 141 572 0125
Fax + 44 (0) 141 572 0246
Email: scotland@mhf.org.uk
UK charity working in mental health and learning disabilities.

Mind

Granta House
15-19 Broadway
Stratford
London
E15 4BQ
Tel: + 44 (0) 20 8519 2122
Mind Information Line: + 44 (0) 20 8522 1728 (if you live in Greater London) or + 44 (0) 8457 660 163 (if you live elsewhere) (9.15am-4.45pm Mon, Wed & Thur)
Email: contact@mind.org.uk
http://www.mind.org.uk

Mental-health charity in England and Wales. Campaigns on behalf of those suffering all types of mental distress (including the Mind model for choice in primary care campaign). Also offers information (via the Mindinfoline and various publications) and support, including counselling, befriending, advocacy, employment and training schemes, and supported housing.

The Samaritans

10 The Grove
Slough
Berks
SL1 1QP
National helpline: + 44 (0) 345 909090
http://www.samaritans.org.uk

UK Helpline for anyone experiencing emotional distress. Someone to talk to in confidence 24 hours a day. Details of local branches can be found in a local telephone directory.

SANE
2nd Floor
Worthington House
199–205 Old Marylebone Road
London
NW1 5QP
Tel: + 44 (0) 20 7375 1002 (office)
Saneline: + 44 (0) 845 767 8000 (open from 12 noon until 2am every day of
the year)
http://www.sane.org.uk
   A campaigning mental health charity. SANELINE is a helpline, giving
information and support to anyone coping with mental illness.

Mental Health Ireland
Mensana House,
6 Adelaide Street
Dun Laoghaire,
Co. Dublin
Tel: 01-2841166
Fax: 01-2841736
Email: info@mentalhealthireland.ie
http://www.mensana.org/
   Voluntary organization aiming to actively support mental health via
advocacy and a range of services and projects (most via affiliate
organizations).

Praxis Mental Health
143 University Street
Belfast
BT7 1HP
Tel: 028 9023 4555
   Provides support services for sufferers from mental illness in Northern
Ireland.

Scottish Association for Mental Health
Cumbrae House
15 Carlton Court
Glasgow
G5 9JP
Tel: +44 (0) 141 568 7000
E-mail: enquire@samh.org.uk
http://www.samh.org.uk

Leading mental-health charity in Scotland. Provides an information service and leaflets on general mental-health issues, as well as running direct services to people with mental-health issues, and campaigning on policy issues.

Stress Watch Scotland
The Barn
42 Barnwell Road
Kilmarnock
KA1 4JF
Tel: + 44 (0) 1563 574144
http://web.ukonline.co.uk/members/stresswatch.scotland/
Provides a helpline for people suffering from stress.

See Me Scotland
http://www.seemescotland.org/
Award-winning Scottish campaign, run by an alliance of five Scottish mental-health organizations (the Highland Users Group, National Schizophrenia Fellowship Scotland, Penumbra, the Royal College of Psychiatrists and the Scottish Association of Mental Health) to deliver Scotland's first national anti-stigma campaign. The 'see me' campaign urges the public to 'see the person not the label', asking them to re-think both their attitudes and their behaviour towards people with a mental-health problem. As well as campaigning to end stigma and raise awareness of mental health, the website lists useful links and sources of further information.

Canadian Mental Health Association (CMHA)
http://www.cmha.ca/
Canadian voluntary organization which aims to promote the mental health of all people and to serve mental-health consumers, their families and friends.

SANE Australia
PO Box 226
South Melbourne 3205
Australia
Tel: +61 3 9682 5933
Fax: +61 3 9682 5944
Email info@sane.org
http://www.sane.org/
National charity helping people affected by mental illness via education, information and campaigns, including StigmaWatch, which monitors the media for content stigmatizing those with mental-health issues.

Carers

Carers' National Association
Tel: 020 8808 7777
Email: info@ukcarers.org
http://www.carersnorth.demon.co.uk

Princess Royal Trust for Carers
Tel: 020 7480 7788
Email: info@carers.org
http://www.carers.org

Depression support and information

Aware
72 Lower Leeson Street
Dublin 2
Eire
Tel: 01 6617211
Fax: 01 6617217
Helpline: 01 6766166
Every day, 10am–10pm
Email: info@aware.ie
http://www.aware.ie/
Voluntary organization aiming to assist those whose lives are directly affected by depression in Ireland.

Depression Alliance
35 Westminster Bridge Road
London
SE1 7JB
Tel: 0207 633 0557
Fax: 0207 633 0559
http://www.depressionalliance.org
Patient self-help group, offering a range of information, including details of local self-help groups. Separate websites for Scotland and Wales branches of the organization. Also offers email support service for members.

Depressives Anonymous
57 Moira Court
Trinity Crescent
London
SW17 7AQ
Tel: 020 8519 1920

Fellowship of Depressives Anonymous
36 Chestnut Avenue
Beverley
North Humberside
HU17 9QU
Main telephone number: 01482 860619
   Supports people suffering from depression on a mutual help basis, complementing professional care. Information service via telephone - 10am–10pm.

Prodigy Guidance on Depression
http://www.prodigy.nhs.uk
   Web site detailing the guidance for NHS GPs in their diagnosis, treatment and management of depression.

Stress, Depression and Anxiety (STAND)
http://www.depression.org.uk/
   Mental-health charity providing a website information resource, with scientific research papers and articles edited to render them understandable to the lay person. Includes a useful glossary of medical terms. Also hosts discussion forums for sufferers to share their experiences, anonymously if desired.

Bipolar disorder
Manic Depression Fellowship
Castle Works
21 St George's Road
London
SE1 6ES
Tel: 020 7793 2600
Fax: 020 7793 2639
Email: mdf@mdf.org.uk
http://www.mdf.org.uk/
   User-led charity organization. Offers a range of self-help resources and support, including a legal-advice line and employment advice.

Depression and Bipolar Support Alliance
Toll free (from within USA): (800) 826-3632
http://www.ndmda.org/
   US patient-led organization.

Organization for Bipolar Affective Disorders Society (OBAD)
1019 – 7th Ave SW
Calgary, Alberta
Canada T2P 1A8
http://www.obad.ca/depressioninfo.htm
Canadian charity based in Calgary for people with bipolar, schizoaffective disorders and unipolar depression. Local support groups and information resources (including 'Ask an expert' facility).

Postnatal depression

Association for Postnatal Illness (APNI)
25 Jerdan Place
Fulham
London
SW6 1BE
Tel: 020 7386 0868
Network of phone and postal volunteers who have had – and recovered from – PND. 24-hour answerphone.

Beyond the Baby Blues
http://www.family-services.org/NewMothers/BeyondBabyBlues.htm
Electronic resource for sufferers of postnatal depression.

Meet-a-Mum Association
26 Avenue Road
London
SE25 4DX
Tel: 020 8771 5595
Postnatal Illness helpline 7pm–10pm: 020 8768 0123
Sufferers from postnatal depression are, where possible, linked with someone local who has suffered from the same problem.

The National Childbirth Trust
Alexander House
Alden Terrace
London
W3 6NH
Tel: 020 8992 8637

Seasonal Affective Disorder

SAD Association
PO Box 989
Steyning

BN44 3HG
http://www.sada.org.uk/
Charity offering advice and support to sufferers.

Bereavement

The Compassionate Friends (TCF)
53 North Street
Bristol
BS3 1EN
Tel: 0117 966 5202
Helpline: 0117 953 9639 (10am–4pm / 6.30pm–10.30pm)
Fax: 0117 914 4368
http://www.tcf.org.uk/
Charity offering local support networks for families who have lost a child.

Cruse Bereavement Care
Cruse House
126 Sheen Road
Richmond
Surrey
TW9 1UR
Tel: 020 8939 9530
Fax: 020 8940 7638
Day by Day Helpline: 0870 167 1677
Email: info@crusebereavementcare.org.uk
http://www.crusebereavementcare.org.uk/
Offers help to anyone who has suffered the loss of a friend or relative. Young person's counsellor available Wednesday, Thursday, Friday (pm) and Saturday.

Foundation for the Study of Infant Deaths
http://www.sids.org.uk

National Association of Bereavement Services
4 Pinchin Street
Shoreditch
London
E1 6DB
Tel: 020 7709 9090

SANDS Stillbirth and Neonatal Death Society
http://www.uk-sands.org

Young people

@ease
c/o Rethink
30 Tabernacle Street
London
EC2A 4DD
Tel: 020 7330 9100
Fax: 020 7330 9102
email: at-ease@rethink.org
Mental health education site aimed at young adults.

Child and Adolescent Bipolar Foundation (CABF)
http://www.bpkids.org/
US not-for-profit organization. Parent-led organization offering information and support for families of sufferers of early-onset bipolar disorder.

ChildLine
Helpline (24 hours): 0800 1111
http://childline.org.uk

Drugs in Schools
388 Old Street
London EC1 9LT
Helpline: 0345 366666

YoungMinds
102–108 Clerkenwell Road
London
EC1M 5SA
Tel: 020 7336 8445
Information line: 0800 018 2138
Fax: 020 7336 8446
http://www.youngminds.org.uk/
Children's mental-health charity. Provides confidential information service, leaflets and consultancy service.

PAPYRUS (Prevention of Suicides)
Rossendale GH
Union Road
Rawtenstall
Lancs BB4 6NE

Email: infoweb1@papyrus-uk.org
http://www.papyrus-uk.org/
　　Organization founded by parents to prevent teenage suicide and raise awareness.

Anti-bullying campaign
Email: help@bullying.co.uk
http://www.bullying.co.uk/
　　Charity which offers advice for pupils, their parents and legal advice.

Anti-Bullying Network
Moray House Institute of Education
University of Edinburgh
Holyrood Road
Edinburgh
EH8 8AQ
Email: abn@mhie.ac.uk
InfoLine: 0131 651 6100
http://www.antibullying.net/

Older people
Age Concern
http://www.ageconcern.org.uk/
　　Charity providing help and practical support for older people. Website gives contact details for regional offices England, Scotland, Wales and N Ireland.

Help the Aged
http://www.helptheaged.org.uk/

Alcohol, addiction and dual-diagnosis issues
Alcohol Concern
http://www.alcoholconcern.org.uk/
　　Website provides a wide range of information, including specific advice for primary care and on dual-diagnosis issues, with a comprehensive list of local groups and information sources.

Alcoholics Anonymous
National Helpline: 0845 76 97 555
http://www.alcoholics-anonymous.org.uk/
　　Support group for alcoholics.

Al-Anon Family Groups (UK and Eire)
61 Great Dover Street
London
SE1 4YF
Tel: 020 7403 0888
Fax: 020 7378 9910
http://www.al-anonuk.org.uk
Support group for family and friends of alcoholics.

Drinkline
1st Floor, 8 Matthew Street
Liverpool
L2 6RE
Tel: 0151 227 4150 (office)
Fax: 0151 227 4019
Email: mmclean@healthwise.org.uk
Helpline: 0800 917 8282 Open Monday to Friday 9am–11pm and Saturday and Sunday 6pm–11pm
Information and advice on sensible drinking and alcohol misuse.

The National Association for Children of Alcoholics
PO Box 64
Fishponds
Bristol
BS16 2UH
Tel: 0117 924 8005
Fax: 0117 942 2928
Helpline: 0800 358 3456
http://www.nacoa.org.uk/

Dual Recovery Anonymous
http://www.draonline.org/
Independent, non-profit, non-professional self-help organization based on 12-step principle.

ADFAM National Helpline
Waterbridge House
32–36 Loman Street
London
SE1 0EE
Tel: 020 7928 8900
Fax: 020 7928 8923
Helpline for the families and friends of drug users.

Narcotics Anonymous (UK region)
UK Service Office
202 City Road
London
EC1V 2PH
Tel: 020 7251 4007
Fax: 020 7251 4006
Email: ukso@ukna.org
UK Helpline: 020 7730 0009
http://www.ukna.org/

Narcotics Anonymous (Ireland)
Helpline Numbers:
Eastern Area: 086-8629308
Southern Area: (021)-278411
Western Area: 086-8149004
Northern Area: 02-890-593636
http://www.na.ireland.org/

References, collected resources and internet portals

DSM Criteria
http://www.psychnet-uk.com

National framework/national guidelines
http://www.doh.gov.uk/nsf/mentalhealth.htm

World Health Report 2001: Mental health: new understanding, new hope
http://www.who.int/whr/2001//main/en/index.htm

NHS Direct
http://www.nhsdirect.nhs.uk/resourceindex.asp

BMJ collected articles
http://bmj.com/cgi/collection/mood_disorders

BBC health site resources
http://www.bbc.co.uk/health/mental/disorders_depression.shtml

Netdoctor
http://depression.netdoctor.co.uk
    Discussion boards, 'ask the expert' and news bulletins. Community developed in association with the Newcastle Affective Disorders Group at University of Newcastle.

Doctor's guide
http://www.docguide.com
US website which gathers latest medical news and information for patients or friends/parents of patients diagnosed with depression.

dotCOMsense
http://www.dotcomsense.com/index.html
The American Psychological Association (APA) website giving information on how to assess mental-health information on the Internet.

Connects
http://www.Connects.org.uk
Free portal to mental health websites run by the Mental Health Foundation (UK). Registration required.

Mental help net
http://mentalhelp.net/
US 'megasite'.

Internet mental health
http://www.mentalhealth.com/
Canadian site of links to resources on various disorders – details on diagnosis, description (European, US), recent research, booklets and links to external sources of information.

British Wheel of Yoga
http://shrewsbury.dsvr.co.uk

Yoga for Health Foundation
http://www.yogaforhealthfoundation.co.uk

Transcendental Meditation
FREEPOST
London SW1P 4YY
Tel: 0800 269303

The Patients Association
http://www.patients-association.com
Includes an index of links to many other patient-directed and information sites.

Patient UK
http://www.patient.co.uk/selfhelp/addict.htm

Counselling

British Association for Counselling and Psychotherapy
1 Regent Place
Rugby
Warwickshire
CV21 2PJ
Tel: +44 (0) 870 443 5252
Fax: +44 (0) 870 443 5160
Email: bac@bac.co.uk
http://www.bac.co.uk/

British Association of Psychotherapists
Tel: 020 8452 9823
http://www.bap-psychotherapy.org/
    Publishes a leaflet *Finding a Therapist.*

British Confederation of Psychotherapists
37 Mapesbury Road
London
NW2 4HJ
Tel: 0208 830 5173
Fax: 0208 452 3684
Email: mail@bcp.org.uk
http://www.bcp.org.uk/

United Kingdom Council for Psychotherapy
http://www.psychotherapy.org.uk/

British Psychoanalytical Society
Tel: 020 7563 5000
http://www.psychoanalysis.org.uk

Drugline Ltd
National helpline: 020 8692 4975
    Freephone Drugline – Dial 100 and ask operator for Freephone Drugline

Marriage Care (formerly Catholic Marriage Advisory Council)
http://marriagecare.org.uk

National Retreat Association
24 South Audley Street
London W1Y 5DL
Tel: 020 7493 3534

One Parent Families
255 Kentish Town Road
London NW5 2LX
Tel: 020 7428 5400
Fax: 020 7482 4851
E-mail: info@oneparentfamilies.org.uk
http://www.oneparentfamilies.org.uk

Relate
11 Little Church Street,
Rugby, Warks CV21 3AP
Tel: 01788 565 675
Email: rugbyrelate@tesco.net
http://www.relate.org.uk

Release
Helpline (10am to 6pm): 020 7729 5255; Overnight 020 7603 8654

Society of Analytical Psychology
Tel: 020 7435 7696
http://www.jungian-analysis.org

Westminster Pastoral Foundation
Tel: 020 7361 4800
http://www.wpf.org

Women's Aid
PO Box 391
Bristol BS99 7WS
Tel: 0117 944 4411
Helpline (24 hours): 0808 2000 246
http://www.womensaid.org.uk

Confederation of Scottish Counselling Agencies
18 Viewfield Street
Stirling
FK8 1UA
Tel: 01786 475140
Fax: 01786 446207
http://www.cosca.org.uk/

Irish Association for Counselling and Therapy
8 Cumberland Street
Dun Laoghaire
Co Dublin
Eire
http://www.irish-counselling.ie/

New Zealand Association of Counsellors
National Office
PO Box 165
Hamilton
2015
New Zealand
http://www.nzac.org.nz/

American Counseling Association
5999 Stevenson Avenue
Alexandria
Virginia 22304-3300
USA
http://www.counseling.org/

Canadian Counselling Association
Suite 702 – 116 Albert Street
Ottawa
Ontario
K1P 5G3
http://www.ccacc.ca/

CBT
Association for Advancement of Behavior Therapy
http://www.aabt.org/
   Professional, interdisciplinary organization serving as a centralized resource and network for behaviour therapy and cognitive behaviour therapy, based in New York, USA.

Clinical trials
Centre for evidence-based mental health
http://www.cebmh.com/
   Evidence-based mental health site.

Emory Clinical Trials

http://www.emoryclinicaltrials.com/

Web site for the mood and anxiety disorders clinical trials at Emory University in Atlanta, GA, USA. Offers listings of current research trials being performed at Emory University for major depression, panic disorder, social phobia, OCD, generalized anxiety disorder, and PTSD.

Harvard Bipolar Research Program

http://www.manicdepressive.org/

Information on current trials, as well as resources for patients and professionals, including clinical tools like mood charts and self-report forms to download.

Mental Health Act

HyperGUIDE

http://www.hyperguide.co.uk/mha

A guide to the Mental Health Act, recommended by the Royal College of Psychiatrists.

The Mental Health Act Commission

http://www.mhac.trent.nhs.uk

A guide to the Mental Health Act, recommended by the Royal College of Psychiatrists.

Electronic media

Coping with Depression (*a learning tape audio pack for the general public published by the Royal College of Psychiatrists*)
http://www.rcpsych.ac.uk/publications/auvideo/depression.htm

Using the Mental Health Act 1997 (*video training resource for doctors, available from the Royal College of Psychiatrists*)
http://www.rcpsych.ac.uk/publications/gaskell/09_9.htm

BIBLIOGRAPHY

JOURNALS

Baldwin, R., Wild, R. Management of depression in later life. *Advances in Psychiatric Treatment*, 2004; 10:131–139

Bhugra, D., Mastrogianni, A. Globalisation and mental disorders: overview with relation to depression. *British Journal of Psychiatry*, 2004; 184:10–20

Carney, R.M., Freedland, K.E. Depression, mortality and medical morbidity in patients with coronary heart disease. *Biological Psychiatry*, 2003; 54:241–247

Cox. J., Holden, J., Sagovsky, R. Detection of postnatal depression. Development of the 10-item Edinburgh Postnatal Depression Scale. *British Journal of Psychiatry*, 1987; 150:782–786.

Editorial. Mood disturbances and coronary heart disease: progress in the past decade. *Medical Journal of Australia*, 2000; 172:151–152

Folstein, M.F., Folstein, S.E., McHugh, P.R. Mini-mental state examination. *Journal of Psychiatric Research*, 1975; 12:189–198

Gilbody, S., House, A.O., Sheldon, T.A. Outcomes research in mental health. Systematic review. *British Journal of Psychiatry*, 2002; 181:8–16

Gilbody, S., Whitty, P. Improving the delivery and organisation of mental health services: beyond the conventional randomised controlled trial. *British Journal of Psychiatry*, 2002, 180:13–18

Hippisley-Cox, J., Fielding, K., Pringle, M. Depression as a risk factor for ischaemic heart disease in men: population based case-control study. *BMJ*, 1998; 316:1714–1719

Jiang, W., Babyak, M.A., Rozanski, A. et al. Depression and increased myocardial ischemic activity in patients with ischemic heart disease. *American Heart Journal*, 2003; 146:55–61

Kessing, L.V. Severity of depressive episodes according to ICD-10: prediction of risk of relapse and suicide. *British Journal of Psychiatry*, 2004; 184:153–156

Montgomery, C. Role of dynamic group therapy in psychiatry. *Advances in Psychiatric Treatment*, 2002; 8:34–41

Smith, D.J., Blackwood, D.H.R. Depression in young adults. *Advances in Psychiatric Treatment*, 2004; 10:4–12

Stores, G. Misdiagnosing sleep disorders as primary psychiatric conditions. *Advances in Psychiatric Treatment*, 2003; 9:69–77

Watkins, E. Combining cognitive therapy with medication in bipolar disorder. *Advances in Psychiatric Treatment*, 2003; 9:110–116

Williams, C. Use of written cognitive–behavioural therapy self-help materials to treat depression. *Advances in Psychiatric Treatment*, 2001; 7:233–240

BOOKS

American Psychiatric Association. Diagnosis and statistical manual of mental disorders, 4th edn. Washington: American Psychiatric Association, 1994

Bazire, B. Psychotropic drug directory. The professionals' pocket handbook and aide memoire. Salisbury: Fivepin Ltd, 2003

Blackburn, I.M. Coping with depression. Edinburgh: Chambers, 1994

British National Formulary, BNF47. London: Pharmaceutical Press, 2004

Burns, D.D. The feeling good handbook: using the new mood therapy in everyday life. New York: Plume Books, 1990

Butler, G., Hope, T. Manage your mind: the

mental fitness guide. Oxford: Oxford University Press, 1996

Down on the farm – coping with depression in rural areas – a farmer's guide. (Available from Health Literature Helpline on 0800 555 777)

Gastpar, M., Kielholz, P. Problems of psychiatry in general practice. Cambridge, MA: Hogrefe and Huber, 1993

Gilbert, P. Overcoming depression: a self-help guide using cognitive behavioural techniques. London: Robinson, 2000.

McConnell, D., Paton, C., Taylor, D., Kerwin, R. The Bethlem and Maudsley NHS Trust: Maudsley prescribing guidelines, 7th edn. London: Taylor and Francis, 2003

Padesky, C., Greenberger, D. The clinician's guide to mind over mood. London: Guildford, 1995

Pitt, B. Down with gloom! or how to defeat depression. London: Gaskell, 1993

Priest, R.G. Anxiety and depression – practical guide to recovery. London: Vermilion, 1996

Rosenthal, N.E. Winter blues – seasonal affective disorder. What it is and how to overcome it. London: Guilford, 1993

Rowe, D. Depression – the way out of your prison, 2nd edn. London: Routledge, 1996

Royal College of Psychiatrists. Psychiatry and general practice today. London: Gaskell, 1994

Shreeve, C. Overcoming depression. London: Thorsons, 1984

Weekes, C. Peace from nervous suffering. London: Thorsons, 1995

Weekes, C. Self help for your nerves London: Thorsons, 1995

World Health Organization. International statistical classification of disease and related health problems, 10th edn. Geneva: WHO, 1992

World Health Organization. The ICD10 classification of mental and behavioural disorders: clinical description and diagnostic guidelines. Geneva: WHO, 1992

ABBREVIATIONS

ADHD – attention deficit hyperactivity disorder
CAT – cognitive and analytical therapy
CBT – cognitive behavioural therapy
CPN – Community Psychiatric Nurse
CSM – Committee on Safety of Medicines
CVA – cerebrovascular accident
DSH – deliberate self-harm
DSM-IV – *Diagnostic and Statistical Manual of Mental Disorders*, 4th edn, published by the American Psychiatric Association
GAD – generalized anxiety disorder
GDS – Geriatric Depression Rating Scale
GHQ – General Health Questionnaire
HADS – Hospital Anxiety and Depression Scale
HRT – hormone replacement therapy
ICD-10 – *International Classification of Diseases*, 10th edn, published by the World Health Organization

MAO(A) – monoamine oxidase-A
MAO(B) – monoamine oxidase-B
MAOI – monoamine oxidase inhibitor
MMSE – Mini-Mental-State Examination
NaRI – noradrenaline reuptake inhibitor
NaSSA – noradrenergic and specific serotonergic antidepressant
OCD – obsessive compulsive disorder
PMT – premenstrual tension
PTSD – post-traumatic shock disorder
RIMA – reversible inhibitor of monoamine oxidase-A
SAD – seasonal affective disorder
SNRI – selective serotonin–noradrenergic reuptake inhibitor
SSRI – selective serotonin reuptake inhibitor
TA – transactional analysis
TCA – tricyclic antidepressant

LIST OF PATIENT QUESTIONS

INDEX

Notes: As depression is the subject of this book, all index entries refer to depression unless otherwise indicated. Entries have been kept to a minimum under 'depression' and readers are advised to seek more specific entries. Page numbers in **bold** refer to figures/tables/boxes.
Abbreviations: CBT, cognitive behavioural therapy; MAOIs, monoamine oxidase inhibitors; NaSSA, noradrenergic and specific serotonergic antidepressants; SSRIs, selective serotonin reuptake inhibitors; TCA, tricyclic antidepressants.

A

E